THE LOW-FODMAP DIET COOKBOOK FOR BEGINNERS

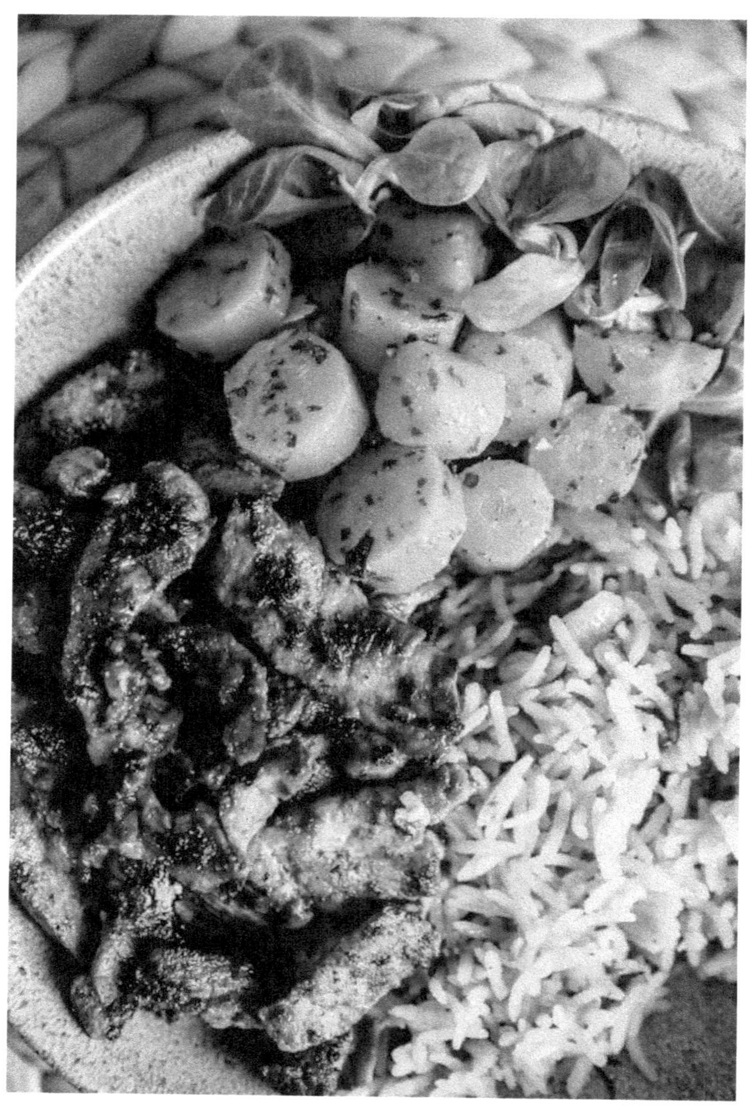

THE LOW-FODMAP DIET COOKBOOK FOR BEGINNERS

Relieve Bloat & IBS, Soothe Your Gut Disorders With This Fast Healthy Recipes

Sabestian Gastronom

BOOKS BY THE AUTHOR

The Complete Mediterranean Diet Cookbook For Beginners

The Complete Plant-Based Diet Cookbook

The Anti-inflammatory Diet Kitchen Cookbook For Beginners

Intermittent Fasting For Women Over

Keto Crockpot Recipes Cookbook

The Complete Slow Cooker Cookbook

The Super Easy Heart-healthy Cookbook

Dash Diet Cookbook

Low Cholesterol Cookbook For Beginners

Intermittent Fasting For Women

To my cherished loved ones,

This cookbook is a labor of love inspired by each one of you who has been a beacon of support and understanding on my journey with a low FODMAP diet. Your unwavering encouragement, patience, and willingness to embrace this lifestyle with me have made the challenges more bearable and the triumphs all the more sweet.

To my family, whose kitchen conversations and shared meals have been the heart of our connection, thank you for adapting and experimenting alongside me. Your willingness to explore new flavors and ingredients has turned our dining table into a space filled with joy and laughter.

To my friends, whose gatherings and celebrations have been marked by thoughtful consideration of my dietary needs, your kindness and consideration have made every social occasion a true celebration of friendship.

To my partner, whose love and support have been a constant source of strength, you have turned what could have been a solitary journey into a shared adventure. Your willingness to explore the world of low FODMAP cuisine with me has made every meal a celebration of our togetherness.

TABLE OF CONTENT

FOREWORD

In the early 2000s, Shepherd and Gibson embarked on groundbreaking research to understand the impact of specific carbohydrates on individuals with irritable bowel syndrome (IBS) and other functional gut disorders. Their studies revealed that certain types of carbohydrates, collectively known as FODMAPs, were poorly absorbed in the small intestine and subsequently fermented by bacteria in the gut. This fermentation process could lead to the production of gas and other byproducts, triggering symptoms such as bloating, abdominal pain, and altered bowel habits in susceptible individuals.

Building on their findings, Shepherd and Gibson developed the low FODMAP diet as a therapeutic approach for managing symptoms associated with IBS and other gastrointestinal conditions. The diet involves restricting the intake of high-FODMAP foods during an initial phase, followed by a systematic reintroduction process to identify specific triggers for each individual. The goal is to create a customized, sustainable dietary plan that minimizes symptomatology while maintaining nutritional adequacy.

INTRODUCTION

This cookbook is a treasury of flavorful recipes meticulously designed to adhere to the principles of the low FODMAP diet. From appetizers to main courses, desserts to beverages, each dish is a testament to the belief that restriction need not equate to blandness. Drawing inspiration from a diverse array of cuisines, the recipes here offer a delightful fusion of taste, texture, and nutritional balance, ensuring that your journey towards digestive wellness is as enjoyable as it is nourishing.

Navigating the low FODMAP landscape involves understanding which fermentable carbohydrates may trigger symptoms. To simplify this process, the cookbook provides a comprehensive list of high and low FODMAP foods, empowering you to make informed choices and create a customized meal plan tailored to your unique needs.

As the author of this cookbook, my commitment to the low FODMAP diet is rooted in personal experience. Like many others, I grappled with the challenges of IBS, searching for a solution that would offer relief without compromising my love for good food. The discovery of the low FODMAP approach was a revelation. It not only transformed my relationship with food but also provided a roadmap to navigate social gatherings and daily meals without fear of digestive distress.

Beyond my own journey, I have had the privilege of witnessing the positive impact of the low FODMAP diet on a diverse range of individuals. From friends and family members to clients and support group participants, the stories are as varied as the recipes in this cookbook. This collection is dedicated to everyone who has embarked on this path towards digestive wellness, seeking not just sustenance but a celebration of flavor, connection, and joy.

The low FODMAP journey is dynamic, and ongoing research continues to refine our understanding of dietary triggers and solutions. With the support of resources like the Monash University Low FODMAP Diet app and a growing community of individuals committed to sharing insights and recipes, the landscape is evolving. This cookbook is a snapshot of the delicious possibilities that exist within the realm of low FODMAP living, and it invites you to join the vibrant community of individuals fostering digestive health and culinary creativity.

As you turn the pages and embark on your own low FODMAP adventure, may these recipes become a source of inspiration, empowerment, and joy. Here's to savoring the flavors of well-being!

CHAPTER 1: UNDERSTANDING LOW_FODMAP DIET

The Low FODMAP (Fermentable Oligosaccharides, Disaccharides, Monosaccharides, and Polyols) diet is a dietary approach designed to manage symptoms of irritable bowel syndrome (IBS) and other gastrointestinal disorders. Developed by researchers at Monash University in Australia, the diet focuses on reducing the intake of specific types of carbohydrates that can trigger digestive symptoms in some individuals.

Short-chain carbohydrates known as FODMAPs are not well absorbed in the small intestine. When they get to the colon, bacteria may ferment them, producing gas and, in those with sensitive digestive systems, causing symptoms including bloating, abdominal pain, diarrhea, and constipation.

There are three primary stages to the Low FODMAP diet:

Elimination Phase:

- During this phase, individuals eliminate high FODMAP foods from their diet for a specific period, typically 2-6 weeks.

- High FODMAP foods include certain fruits (e.g., apples, cherries, watermelon), vegetables (e.g., onions, garlic, cauliflower), legumes, certain grains, dairy products containing lactose, and certain sweeteners (e.g., sorbitol, mannitol).

- The goal is to give the gut a chance to settle and alleviate symptoms.

Reintroduction Phase:

- In this phase, specific FODMAPs are gradually reintroduced one at a time to identify which ones trigger symptoms in individual cases.

- This phase helps determine personal tolerance levels and allows for a more personalized and varied diet.

Maintenance Phase:

- Based on the results of the reintroduction phase, individuals can establish a long-term, sustainable diet that minimizes symptoms while allowing for a variety of foods.

- Some people may need to continue avoiding certain high FODMAP foods, while others may tolerate them in moderation.

It's important to note that the Low FODMAP diet is not a one-size-fits-all approach, and guidance from a registered dietitian or healthcare professional is recommended. Additionally, the diet should not be followed without supervision, as it can be restrictive and may lead to nutritional deficiencies if not implemented correctly.

Key points to understand about the Low FODMAP diet:

- It is not a lifelong diet but rather a diagnostic and therapeutic tool.
- It aims to identify and reduce specific carbohydrates that can trigger digestive symptoms.
- The diet is individualized, and the reintroduction phase helps determine personal tolerance levels.
- Professional guidance is crucial to ensure nutritional adequacy and overall well-being while following the diet.

Benefits of Low FODMAP Cooking

Engaging in low FODMAP cooking can offer several potential benefits for individuals with irritable bowel syndrome (IBS) or other digestive issues. Here are some of the advantages associated with adopting a low FODMAP approach in cooking:

Symptom Management for IBS: The primary purpose of the low FODMAP diet is to alleviate symptoms associated with IBS, such as bloating, gas, abdominal pain, and changes in bowel habits. By avoiding high-FODMAP foods, individuals may experience a reduction in these symptoms.

Personalized Approach: The low FODMAP diet is not a one-size-fits-all solution. Through a structured reintroduction phase, individuals can identify specific FODMAPs that trigger their symptoms, allowing for a more personalized and sustainable long-term eating plan.

Improved Quality of Life: For those with IBS, managing symptoms effectively can significantly improve their overall quality of life. Reduced digestive discomfort can lead to better physical and emotional well-being.

Nutrient Intake Awareness: Following a low FODMAP diet requires careful attention to food choices. This heightened awareness often leads individuals to become more conscious of their nutrient intake, promoting a balanced and healthful diet.

Diverse Culinary Exploration: While certain high-FODMAP foods are restricted, there is still a wide variety of low-FODMAP ingredients available. This can encourage individuals to explore and experiment with different foods, flavors, and cooking techniques to create enjoyable and satisfying meals.

Increased Confidence in Food Choices: Knowing which foods are low in FODMAPs and well-tolerated can empower individuals to make more confident food choices, both at home and when dining out. This can be especially beneficial in social situations where food choices may be limited.

Potential Weight Management: Some individuals find that adhering to a low FODMAP diet helps with weight management. However, it's essential to approach this aspect with caution and ensure that the diet remains balanced and nutritionally adequate.

Reduced Dependency on Medications: For some individuals, effective management of IBS symptoms through dietary modifications may lead to a decreased reliance on medications to control digestive issues.

It's crucial to note that the low FODMAP diet should be undertaken under the guidance of a healthcare professional, typically a registered dietitian, to ensure proper implementation, nutritional adequacy, and long-term well-being. The diet is not suitable for everyone, and its effectiveness can vary from person to person.

Tips for Successful Low FODMAP Meal Preparation

Successfully preparing low FODMAP meals involves careful planning, ingredient selection, and attention to portion sizes. Here are some tips to help you navigate and enjoy your low FODMAP meal preparation:

Educate Yourself: Familiarize yourself with the list of high and low FODMAP foods. Refer to reputable resources or work with a registered dietitian who specializes in the low FODMAP diet to ensure accuracy.

Plan Your Meals: Plan your meals in advance to ensure a variety of flavors and nutrients. This will also help you avoid last-minute decisions that may lead to inadvertently consuming high-FODMAP foods.

Explore Low FODMAP Ingredients: Get creative with low FODMAP ingredients such as rice, quinoa, potatoes, meats, poultry, fish, eggs, lactose-free dairy, and a variety of fruits and vegetables that are low in FODMAPs.

Experiment with Herbs and Spices: Herbs and spices can add flavor to your meals without introducing high FODMAP ingredients. Experiment with garlic-infused oils, as they can provide a garlic flavor without the FODMAP content.

Batch Cooking: Consider batch cooking and preparing meals in advance to save time during the week. This can be especially helpful when adhering to a restrictive diet.

Read Labels: Be diligent about reading food labels, as some processed foods may contain hidden high-FODMAP ingredients. Pay attention to additives, sweeteners, and preservatives.

Mind Portion Sizes: Pay attention to portion sizes, especially when it comes to certain fruits, vegetables, and grains. Consuming large amounts of even low FODMAP foods can contribute to symptoms.

Use Low FODMAP Substitutes: Explore low FODMAP alternatives for common ingredients. For example, use lactose-free dairy, gluten-free flours, and alternative sweeteners like maple syrup or stevia.

Experiment with Cooking Techniques: Try different cooking techniques such as grilling, roasting, or sautéing to enhance flavors without relying on high FODMAP ingredients.

Keep a Food Diary: Keep a food diary to track your meals and any symptoms you may experience. This can help you identify patterns and refine your low FODMAP approach over time.

Stay Hydrated: Drink plenty of water throughout the day to stay hydrated, which is important for overall well-being and digestive health.

Be Flexible and Patient: The low FODMAP diet can be challenging at first, but be patient and flexible as you learn more about your individual tolerances. It's a process of trial and error.

Remember that everyone's tolerance to specific FODMAPs can vary, so what works for one person may not work for another. Consulting with a healthcare professional, particularly a registered dietitian specializing in the low FODMAP diet, can provide personalized guidance and support throughout your journey.

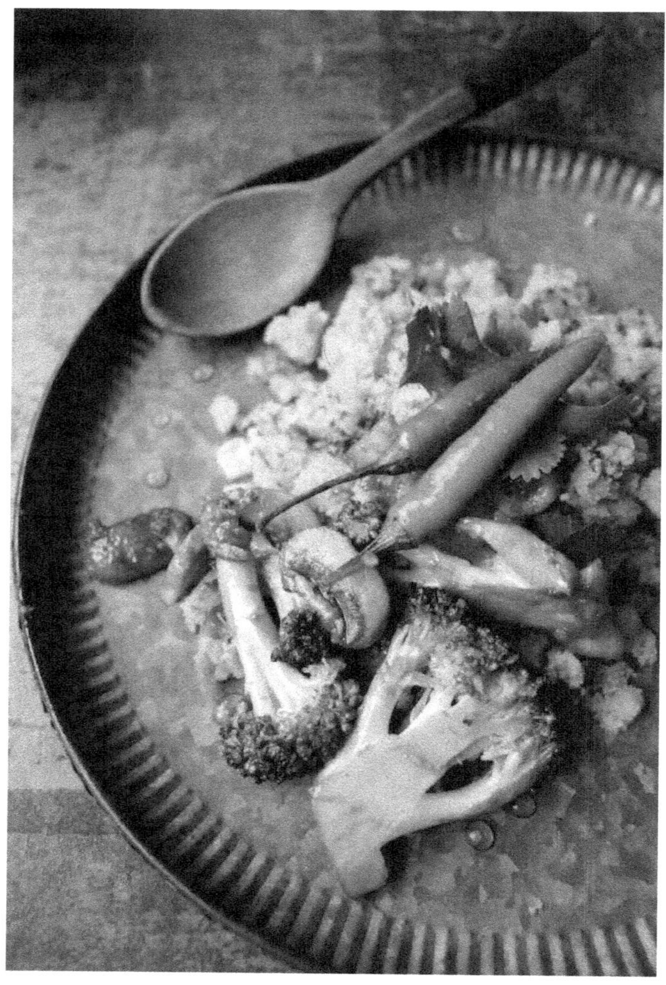

CHAPTER 2:KITCHEN ESSENTIALS FOR LOW FODMAP COOKING

Stocking a Low FODMAP Pantry

Stocking a low-FODMAP pantry involves selecting foods that are low in fermentable carbohydrates, which can be beneficial for individuals with irritable bowel syndrome (IBS) or other digestive issues. FODMAPs (Fermentable Oligosaccharides, Disaccharides, Monosaccharides, and Polyols) are types of carbohydrates that can trigger symptoms in some people.

Here's a guide to stocking a low-FODMAP pantry:

Grains and Cereals:
- Quinoa
- Rice (white and brown)
- Oats (gluten-free)
- Polenta (cornmeal)

Proteins:
- Fresh or frozen meats (chicken, beef, pork, lamb)

- Fresh or frozen fish and seafood
- Eggs
- Tofu

Canned and Packaged Goods:
- Canned tomatoes (in moderation)
- Canned tuna (in water)
- Canned salmon
- Olives
- Pickles (without high-FODMAP ingredients)
- Canned chickpeas (drained and rinsed)

Dairy and Alternatives:
- Lactose-free milk or almond milk
- Hard cheeses (cheddar, Swiss, mozzarella)
- Butter (lactose-free if needed)
- Lactose-free yogurt

Fruits (in moderation):
- Berries (strawberries, blueberries, raspberries)
- Cantaloupe
- Grapes
- Kiwi
- Pineapple

Vegetables:
- Carrots
- Bell peppers
- Zucchini
- Cucumbers
- Leafy greens (spinach, kale, lettuce)

Nuts and Seeds (in moderation):

- Almonds (limited to a small serving)
- Walnuts (limited to a small serving)
- Chia seeds
- Sunflower seeds

Baking Supplies:

- flour (rice flour, potato flour) devoid of gluten
- Baking powder (check for additives)
- Vanilla extract
- Dark chocolate (low-FODMAP)

Condiments and Sauces:

- Olive oil
- Vinegar (balsamic in small amounts)
- Mustard
- Mayonnaise (without high-FODMAP ingredients)
- Soy sauce (use tamari for a gluten-free option)

Herbs and Spices:

- Basil
- Oregano
- Rosemary
- Thyme
- Cumin
- Ginger (fresh or ground)

Remember to check ingredient labels for hidden sources of high-FODMAP ingredients. Additionally, serving sizes can impact FODMAP content, so it's essential to be mindful of portions. If you have specific dietary requirements or restrictions, it's advisable to consult with a healthcare professional or a registered dietitian for personalized guidance.

Essential Low FODMAP Cooking Tools

The Low FODMAP (Fermentable Oligosaccharides, Disaccharides, Monosaccharides, and Polyols) diet is often recommended for individuals with irritable bowel syndrome (IBS) or other digestive disorders. When following a Low FODMAP diet, it's important to have the right cooking tools to make meal preparation easier. Here are some essential low FODMAP cooking tools:

Food Scale:

- A digital kitchen scale is crucial for accurately measuring ingredients. This is important when following specific serving sizes of low FODMAP foods.

Measuring Cups and Spoons:

- Have a set of measuring cups and spoons for precise measuring of ingredients, especially when working with small amounts.

FODMAP-Friendly Recipe Book or App:

- Invest in a cookbook or use a mobile app that focuses on low FODMAP recipes. This will help you plan meals that adhere to the dietary restrictions.

Non-Stick Cookware:

- Non-stick pots and pans are helpful for cooking without excessive amounts of added fats or oils. This can be important for individuals with sensitive digestive systems.

Vegetable Peeler:

- A vegetable peeler is useful for peeling and preparing vegetables that are allowed on the low FODMAP diet.

Chef's Knife:

- A good quality chef's knife makes chopping and dicing fruits, vegetables, and meats more efficient.

Herb and Spice Grinder:

- Whole spices and herbs are often preferred on a low FODMAP diet. Having a grinder allows you to use fresh, flavorful options without added fillers.

Colander:

- A colander is handy for draining and rinsing canned goods, such as beans or lentils, to reduce their FODMAP content.

Slow Cooker:

- A slow cooker can be a time-saving tool, allowing you to prepare meals with minimal hands-on time.

Food Storage Containers:

- Have a variety of containers for storing leftovers. This will help you plan and prepare meals in advance, reducing the need for last-minute cooking.

Lactose-Free Dairy Alternatives:

- Depending on your specific dietary needs, you may want to have lactose-free dairy alternatives on hand, such as lactose-free milk or cheese.

Grill or Grill Pan:

- Grilling is a great way to add flavor to meats and vegetables without the need for high-FODMAP marinades or sauces.

Zester:

- A zester is useful for adding citrus flavor to dishes without using high-FODMAP juices

Selecting FODMAP-Friendly Ingredients

When following a Low FODMAP diet, it's essential to choose ingredients that are FODMAP-friendly. Here's a general guide to selecting low FODMAP ingredients for your meals:

Proteins:

- Choose lean meats, poultry, and fish. Avoid processed or cured meats that may contain high-FODMAP additives.

- Eggs are generally well-tolerated.

Vegetables:

- Opt for low FODMAP vegetables such as leafy greens, carrots, bell peppers, zucchini, cucumber, and tomatoes (in moderation).

- Avoid high FODMAP vegetables like onions, garlic, cauliflower, broccoli, and mushrooms.

Fruits:

- Stick to low FODMAP fruits like strawberries, blueberries, kiwi, pineapple, and grapes.

- Limit or avoid high FODMAP fruits such as apples, pears, mangoes, watermelon, and stone fruits.

Grains:

- Opt for grains devoid of gluten, such as corn, rice, quinoa, and oats.

- Be cautious with wheat-based products, as they often contain fructans, a high-FODMAP ingredient.

Dairy and Alternatives:

- Use lactose-free or low-lactose dairy products like lactose-free milk, hard cheeses, and lactose-free yogurt.

- Opt for dairy alternatives like almond milk or coconut milk, ensuring they are free from high-FODMAP additives.

Fats and Oils:

- Most fats and oils are low FODMAP. Use olive oil, canola oil, and other tolerated oils for cooking.

- Be cautious with high-FODMAP additives in some salad dressings and spreads.

Nuts and Seeds:

- Choose low FODMAP nuts and seeds, such as almonds (limited quantity), macadamia nuts, and chia seeds.

- Limit or avoid high FODMAP nuts like cashews and pistachios.

Sweeteners:
- Opt for sweeteners that are low FODMAP, such as glucose, maple syrup, and stevia.
- Steer clear of sweeteners with high fructose corn syrup, agave syrup, and honey content.

Herbs and Spices:
- Most herbs and spices are low FODMAP. Use fresh or dried herbs like basil, oregano, and parsley.
- Limit garlic and onion, substituting with infused oils or garlic-infused oil for flavor.

Beverages:
- Stick to water, herbal teas, and low FODMAP fruit juices in moderation.
- Limit or avoid high FODMAP beverages like regular sodas, high-fructose corn syrup-containing drinks, and some alcoholic beverages.

Always refer to the Monash University Low FODMAP Diet app or other reliable resources for the most up-to-date information on specific foods and their FODMAP content.

CHAPTER 3: BREAKFAST DELIGHTS

Quinoa Breakfast Bowl

Ingredients:
- 1 cup cooked quinoa
- 1/2 cup lactose-free yogurt
- 1/2 cup strawberries, sliced
- 1 tablespoon chia seeds

Preparation:
1. Mix quinoa and yogurt in a bowl.
2. Top with sliced strawberries and sprinkle chia seeds.
3. Serve chilled.

Nutritional Information:
- Calories: 300
- Protein: 12g
- Carbohydrates: 45g
- Fat: 8g

Egg and Spinach Omelet

Ingredients:
- 2 eggs
- 1 cup spinach, chopped
- 1 tablespoon olive oil

- Salt and pepper to taste

Preparation:

1. Whisk eggs and season with salt and pepper.

2. Sauté spinach in olive oil until wilted.

3. Pour eggs over spinach, cook until set, and fold.

Nutritional Information:

- Calories: 250

- Protein: 18g

- Carbohydrates: 2g

- Fat: 18g

Low-FODMAP Smoothie Bowl

Ingredients:

- 1 banana (under-ripe)

- 1/2 cup blueberries

- 1/2 cup lactose-free yogurt

- 1 tablespoon almond butter

Preparation:

1. Blend banana, blueberries, and yogurt until smooth.

2. Pour into a bowl and top with almond butter.

Nutritional Information:

- Calories: 280

- Protein: 8g

- Carbohydrates: 35g

- Fat: 12g

Smoked Salmon and Avocado Toast

Ingredients:
- 2 slices gluten-free bread
- 2 oz smoked salmon
- 1/2 avocado, sliced
- Chives for garnish

Preparation:
1. Toast gluten-free bread.
2. Top with smoked salmon, avocado slices, and garnish with chives.

Nutritional Information:
- Calories: 320
- Protein: 15g
- Carbohydrates: 25g
- Fat: 18g

Peanut Butter Banana Rice Cakes

Ingredients:
- 2 rice cakes
- 2 tablespoons peanut butter
- 1 banana, sliced

Preparation:
1. Spread peanut butter on rice cakes.
2. Top with banana slices.

Nutritional Information:
- Calories: 280
- Protein: 7g
- Carbohydrates: 35g
- Fat: 14g

Chia Seed Pudding

Ingredients:
- 2 tablespoons chia seeds
- 1 cup lactose-free milk
- 1/2 teaspoon vanilla extract
- 1 tablespoon maple syrup

Preparation:
1. Mix chia seeds, milk, vanilla extract, and maple syrup.
2. Refrigerate overnight.
3. Serve with berries.

Nutritional Information:
- Calories: 220
- Protein: 6g
- Carbohydrates: 20g
- Fat: 12g

Feta and Spinach Frittata

Ingredients:
- 4 eggs
- 1 cup spinach, chopped

- 2 oz feta cheese, crumbled
- 1 tablespoon olive oil

Preparation:

1. Sauté spinach in olive oil until wilted.

2. Whisk eggs and pour over spinach.

3. Add feta, cook until set.

Nutritional Information:

- Calories: 280
- Protein: 15g
- Carbohydrates: 3g
- Fat: 22g

Low-FODMAP Pancakes

Ingredients:

- 1 cup gluten-free flour
- 1 tablespoon maple syrup
- 1/2 cup lactose-free milk
- 1 egg

Preparation:

1. Mix flour, maple syrup, milk, and egg.

2. Cook pancakes on a griddle.

Nutritional Information:

- Calories: 240
- Protein: 7g
- Carbohydrates: 40g
- Fat: 6g

Greek Yogurt Parfait

Ingredients:
- 1 cup lactose-free Greek yogurt
- 1/4 cup granola (gluten-free)
- 1/2 cup raspberries

Preparation:
1. Layer yogurt, granola, and raspberries in a glass.

Nutritional Information:
- Calories: 280
- Protein: 15g
- Carbohydrates: 30g
- Fat: 12g

Turkey and Tomato Breakfast Wrap

Ingredients:
- 1 gluten-free tortilla
- 3 oz turkey slices
- 1 tomato, sliced
- Lettuce leaves

Preparation:
1. Lay out the tortilla and layer with turkey, tomato, and lettuce.
2. Roll up into a wrap.

Nutritional Information:

- Calories: 300
- Protein: 20g
- Carbohydrates: 25g
- Fat: 12g

Baked Blueberry Oatmeal Cups

Ingredients:

- 2 cups rolled oats
- 1 cup lactose-free milk
- 1/4 cup maple syrup
- 1/2 cup blueberries

Preparation:

1. Mix oats, milk, and maple syrup.
2. Fold in blueberries and spoon into muffin cups.
3. Bake until set.

Nutritional Information:

- Calories: 220
- Protein: 8g
- Carbohydrates: 35g
- Fat: 6g

Sautéed Zucchini and Eggs

Ingredients:

- 2 eggs
- 1 zucchini, sliced

- 1 tablespoon olive oil
- Salt and pepper to taste

Preparation:

1. Sauté zucchini in olive oil until tender.
2. Crack eggs over zucchini, season with salt and pepper.
3. Cook until eggs are done.

Nutritional Information:

- Calories: 240
- Protein: 12g
- Carbohydrates: 6g
- Fat: 18g

Note: Nutritional information is approximate and may vary based on specific brands and quantities used.

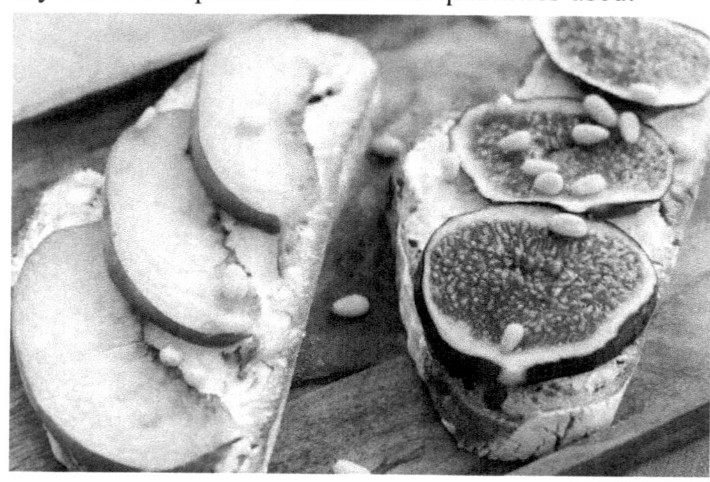

CHAPTER 4: LUNCHTIME FAVORITES

Grilled Chicken Salad

Ingredients:
- 1 boneless, skinless chicken breast
- Mixed salad greens (lettuce, spinach, arugula)
- Cherry tomatoes
- Cucumber slices
- Olive oil
- Lemon juice
- Salt and pepper to taste

Preparation:
1. Season the chicken breast with salt and pepper, then grill until fully cooked.
2. In a bowl, toss salad greens, cherry tomatoes, and cucumber slices.
3. Slice the grilled chicken and place it on top of the salad.
4. Drizzle with olive oil and lemon juice.

Nutritional Information:
Calories: 300-350 | Protein: 30g | Carbohydrates: 10g | Fat: 15g

Quinoa and Veggie Stir-Fry

Ingredients:
- 1 cup cooked quinoa
- Bell peppers (red, yellow, or green)
- Zucchini
- Carrots
- Green beans
- Tamari sauce
- Ginger
- Sesame oil

Preparation:
1. Stir-fry sliced bell peppers, zucchini, carrots, and green beans in sesame oil.
2. Add cooked quinoa to the vegetables.
3. Mix in tamari sauce and grated ginger.
4. Cook until heated through.

Nutritional Information:
Calories: 350-400 | Protein: 12g | Carbohydrates: 50g | Fat: 15g

Turkey and Lettuce Wraps

Ingredients:
- Turkey slices
- Bibb lettuce leaves
- Sliced bell peppers
- Cucumber strips

- Mayonnaise (low FODMAP)

Preparation:

1. Lay out a lettuce leaf and place turkey slices on it.

2. Add bell peppers and cucumber strips.

3. Spread a thin layer of low FODMAP mayonnaise.

4. Roll, then use a toothpick to fasten.

Nutritional Details:

250–300 calories, 20g of protein, 5g of carbohydrates, and 15g of fat.

Baked Salmon with Lemon-Dill Sauce

Ingredients:
- Salmon filet
- Lemon juice
- Fresh dill
- Olive oil
- Salt and pepper

Preparation:

1. Preheat the oven and bake salmon with olive oil, salt, and pepper.

2. Prepare a sauce by mixing lemon juice and chopped dill.

3. Pour the lemon-dill sauce over the baked salmon.

Nutritional Information:

Calories: 350-400 | Protein: 25g | Carbohydrates: 0g | Fat: 20g

Egg Salad Lettuce Wrap

Ingredients:
- Hard-boiled eggs
- Green onions (green parts only)
- Dijon mustard
- Olive oil
- Lettuce leaves

Preparation:
1. Chop hard-boiled eggs and mix with sliced green onions.
2. Add Dijon mustard and olive oil, mixing well.
3. Spoon the egg salad on lettuce leaves and wrap.

Nutritional Information:
Calories: 200-250 | Protein: 15g | Carbohydrates: 5g | Fat: 15g

Shrimp and Vegetable Skewers

Ingredients:
- Shrimp, peeled and deveined
- Cherry tomatoes
- Zucchini chunks
- Bell pepper chunks
- Olive oil
- Lemon zest
- Fresh parsley

Preparation:

1. Thread shrimp, cherry tomatoes, zucchini, and bell peppers onto skewers.

2. Drizzle with olive oil, sprinkle lemon zest and fresh parsley.

3. Grill or broil until shrimp are cooked.

Nutritional Details

250–300 calories, 20g of protein, 10g of carbohydrates, and 15g of fat.

Low FODMAP Sushi Bowl

Ingredients:

- Sushi rice (cooked)
- Sliced cucumber
- Nori seaweed, shredded
- Cooked shrimp or crab
- Soy sauce (low FODMAP)

Preparation:

1. Arrange sushi rice in a bowl.

2. Top with sliced cucumber, shredded nori, and cooked shrimp or crab.

3. Drizzle with low FODMAP soy sauce.

Nutritional Details

300–350 calories, 15g of protein, 60g of carbohydrates, and 5g of fat.

Caprese Salad Skewers

Ingredients:
- Cherry tomatoes
- Fresh mozzarella balls
- Basil leaves
- Balsamic glaze
- Olive oil

Preparation:
1. Thread cherry tomatoes, mozzarella balls, and basil leaves onto skewers.
2. Drizzle with olive oil and balsamic glaze before serving.

Nutritional Information:
Calories: 200-250 | Protein: 10g | Carbohydrates: 5g | Fat: 15g

Spinach and Feta Stuffed Chicken Breast

Ingredients:
- Chicken breast
- Spinach leaves
- Feta cheese (crumbled)
- Lemon zest
- Paprika
- Olive oil

Preparation:

1. Butterfly the chicken breast and stuff with spinach and crumbled feta.
2. Season with lemon zest and paprika.
3. Bake until the chicken is cooked through.

Nutritional Information:

Calories: 300-350 | Protein: 30g | Carbohydrates: 2g | Fat: 15g

Please note that nutritional information is approximate and may vary based on specific ingredients and portion sizes.

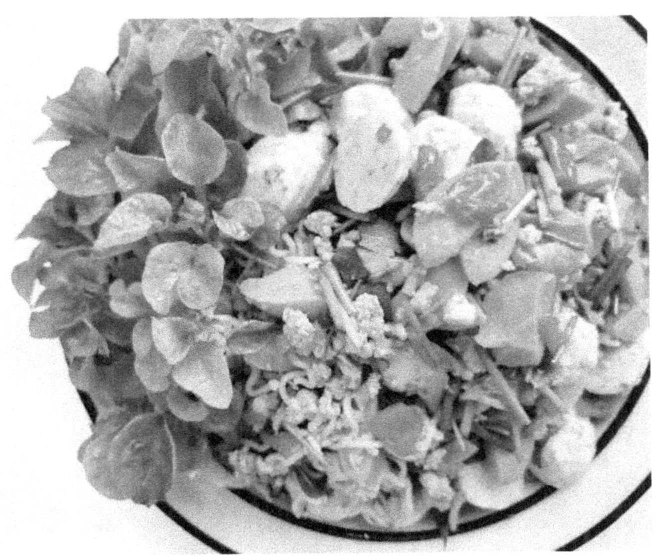

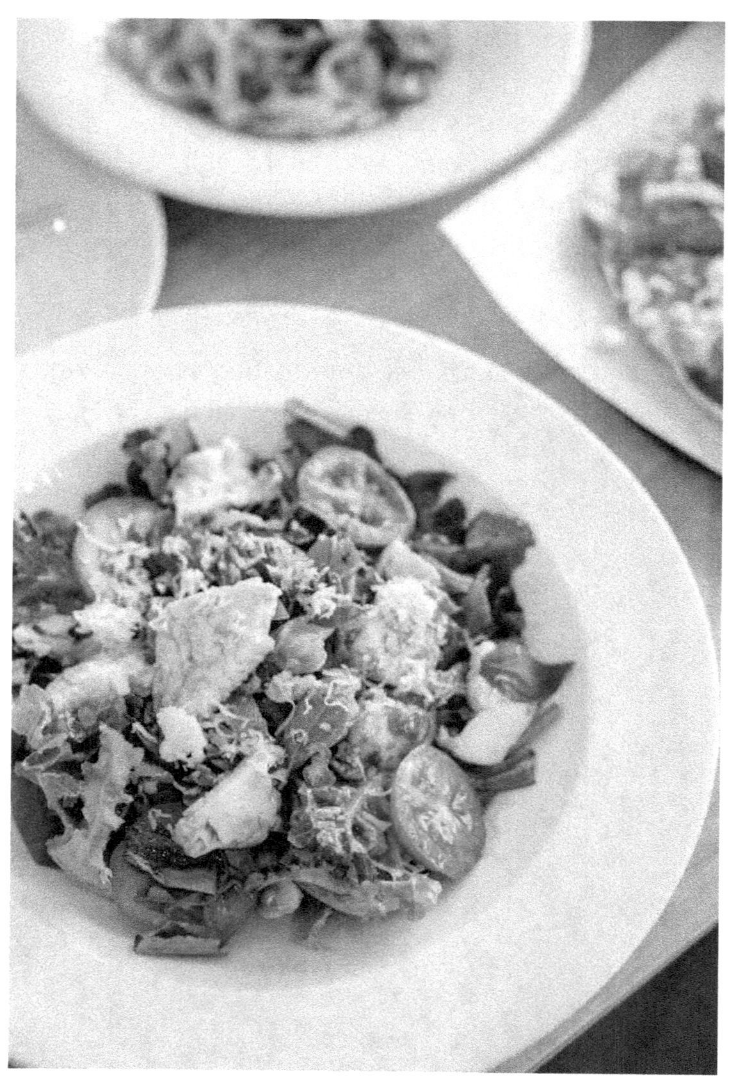

CHAPTER 5: SATISFYING SNACKS

Baked Parmesan Zucchini Chips:

- **Ingredients:**
  - Zucchini
  - Parmesan cheese
  - Olive oil
  - Salt and pepper
- **Preparation:**
  - Set oven temperature to 425°F (220°C).
  - Cut zucchini into slender rounds.
  - Toss with olive oil, and season with salt, pepper, and Parmesan.
  - Bake until crispy, about 15 to 20 minutes.
  - **Nutritional Information (per serving):** Calories: 90, Protein: 5g, Fat: 7g, Carbohydrates: 3g, Fiber: 1g.

Greek Yogurt with Blueberries and Almonds:

- **Ingredients:**
  - Greek yogurt
  - Blueberries
  - Almonds

- **Preparation:**
  - Spoon Greek yogurt into a bowl.
  - Top with fresh blueberries and sliced almonds.
  - **Nutritional Information (per serving):** Calories: 150, Protein: 15g, Fat: 8g, Carbohydrates: 10g, Fiber: 2g.

Peanut butter and banana on rice cake:

- **Ingredients:**
  - Rice cake
  - Peanut butter (ensure no added high-FODMAP ingredients)
  - Banana slices
- **Preparation:**
  - Spread peanut butter on the rice cake.
  - Top with banana slices.
  - **Nutritional Information (per serving):** Calories: 200, Protein: 6g, Fat: 10g, Carbohydrates: 24g, Fiber: 3g.

Cucumber and Smoked Salmon Rolls:

- **Ingredients:**
  - Cucumber

- Smoked salmon
- Cream cheese (lactose-free if necessary)
- **Preparation:**
- Slice cucumbers into thin strips.
- Spread a thin layer of cream cheese on each strip and top with smoked salmon.
- **Nutritional Information (per serving):** Calories: 120, Protein: 15g, Fat: 7g, Carbohydrates: 2g, Fiber: 0g.

Homemade Trail Mix:

- **Ingredients:**
  - Almonds
  - Walnuts
  - Pumpkin seeds
  - Dark chocolate chips
- **Preparation:**
  - Mix equal parts of almonds, walnuts, pumpkin seeds, and dark chocolate chips.
- **Nutritional Information (per serving):** Calories: 180, Protein: 5g, Fat: 15g, Carbohydrates: 10g, Fiber: 3g.

Quinoa Salad Cups:

- **Ingredients:**
  - Quinoa (cooked and cooled)
  - Cherry tomatoes (halved)

- Cucumber (diced)
- Feta cheese (crumbled)
- Lemon juice and olive oil for dressing

Preparation:

- To prepare, combine quinoa, cucumber, cherry tomatoes, and feta cheese.
- Dress with a drizzle of lemon juice and olive oil.
- **Nutritional Information (per serving):** Calories: 220, Protein: 8g, Fat: 12g, Carbohydrates: 20g, Fiber: 3g.

Baked Buffalo Chicken Wings:

- **Ingredients:**
  - Chicken wings
  - Buffalo sauce (check for low-FODMAP ingredients)
  - Olive oil
  - Salt and pepper
- **Preparation:**
  - Preheat the oven to 400°F (200°C).
  - Toss chicken wings with olive oil, salt, and pepper.
  - Bake until crispy, then toss in buffalo sauce.
  - Nutritional Information (per serving): Calories: 250, Protein: 20g, Fat: 18g, Carbohydrates: 2g, Fiber: 0g.

Caprese Skewers:

- **Ingredients:**

- Cherry tomatoes
- Mozzarella balls
- Basil leaves
- Balsamic glaze
- **Preparation:**
  - Attach mozzarella balls, cherry tomatoes, and basil leaves on skewers.
  - Just before serving, drizzle with balsamic glaze.
  - **Nutritional Information (per serving):** Calories: 160, Protein: 10g, Fat: 10g, Carbohydrates: 8g, Fiber: 1g.

Oven-Roasted Chickpeas:

- **Ingredients:**
  - Canned chickpeas (rinsed and dried)
  - Olive oil
  - Cumin, paprika, salt, and pepper (seasonings)
- **Preparation:**
  - Toss chickpeas with olive oil and seasonings.
  - Roast in the oven until crispy.
  - **Nutritional Information (per serving):** Calories: 180, Protein: 8g, Fat: 6g, Carbohydrates: 25g, Fiber: 6g.

Turkey and Lettuce Wraps:

- **Ingredients:**
  - Sliced turkey

- Lettuce leaves
- Mayonnaise (low-FODMAP)
- Tomato slices
- **Preparation:**
  - Spread a thin layer of mayonnaise on a lettuce leaf.
  - Layer with turkey slices and tomato, then wrap.
  - **Nutritional Information (per serving):** Calories: 150, Protein: 15g, Fat: 8g, Carbohydrates: 3g, Fiber: 1g.

Chocolate Chia Seed Pudding:

- **Ingredients:**
  - Chia seeds
  - Almond milk (unsweetened)
  - Cocoa powder
  - Maple syrup (optional)
- **Preparation:**
  - Stir together the chia seeds, almond milk, maple syrup, and chocolate powder. Chill in the fridge for the entire night, or until the pudding consistency is reached.
  - **Nutritional Information (per serving):** Calories: 150, Protein: 5g, Fat: 10g, Carbohydrates: 15g, Fiber: 8g.

Note: Adjust portion sizes and ingredients based on your specific dietary needs and preferences.

CHAPTER 6: DINNER CREATIONS

Grilled Lemon Herb Chicken

Ingredients:
- 4 boneless, skinless chicken breasts
- 2 tablespoons olive oil
- 1 tablespoon fresh lemon juice
- 1 teaspoon dried oregano
- Salt and pepper to taste

Preparation:
1. Preheat the grill to medium-high heat.
2. In a bowl, mix olive oil, lemon juice, oregano, salt, and pepper.
3. Coat chicken breasts with the mixture and grill for 6-8 minutes per side or until fully cooked.

Nutritional Information:
- Calories: 250 per serving
- Protein: 30g
- Fat: 13g
- Carbohydrates: 2g

Quinoa and Roasted Vegetable Salad

Ingredients:
- 1 cup quinoa
- 2 cups mixed low FODMAP vegetables (zucchini, bell peppers, cherry tomatoes)
- 2 tablespoons olive oil
- 1 tablespoon balsamic vinegar
- Salt and pepper to taste

Preparation:
1. Cook quinoa according to package instructions.
2. Toss vegetables in olive oil, roast in the oven at 400°F (200°C) for 20 minutes.
3. Mix cooked quinoa, roasted vegetables, balsamic vinegar, salt, and pepper.

Nutritional Information:
- Calories: 300 per serving
- Protein: 8g
- Fat: 12g
- Carbohydrates: 40g

Shrimp Stir-Fry with Bok Choy

Ingredients:
- 1 lb shrimp, peeled and deveined
- 2 cups bok choy, chopped
- 1 bell pepper, sliced

- 2 tablespoons sesame oil
- 1 tablespoon soy sauce (use gluten-free)

Preparation:

1. Heat sesame oil in a pan, add shrimp, bok choy, and bell pepper.
2. Stir-fry until shrimp are cooked and vegetables are tender.
3. Add soy sauce, toss, and serve.

Nutritional Information:

- Calories: 220 per serving
- Protein: 25g
- Fat: 10g
- Carbohydrates: 6g

Turkey and Quinoa Stuffed Peppers

Ingredients:

- 4 bell peppers, halved and seeds removed
- 1 lb ground turkey
- 1 cup cooked quinoa
- 1 cup diced tomatoes
- 1 teaspoon cumin
- Salt and pepper to taste

Preparation:

1. Preheat the oven to 375°F (190°C).
2. In a skillet, cook ground turkey until browned.

3. Mix cooked turkey with quinoa, diced tomatoes, cumin, salt, and pepper.

4. Stuff the halved peppers with the mixture and bake for 25-30 minutes.

Nutritional Information:

- Calories: 280 per serving
- Protein: 24g
- Fat: 10g
- Carbohydrates: 25g

Salmon with Lemon-Dill Sauce

Ingredients:

- 4 salmon filets
- 2 tablespoons olive oil
- 1 tablespoon fresh dill, chopped
- 1 tablespoon lemon juice
- Salt and pepper to taste

Preparation:

1. Preheat the oven to 400°F (200°C).

2. Place salmon on a baking sheet, drizzle with olive oil, and sprinkle with dill, lemon juice, salt, and pepper.

3. Bake for 15-20 minutes or until salmon is cooked through.

Nutritional Information:

- Calories: 320 per serving
- Protein: 25g
- Fat: 22g

- Carbohydrates: 1g

Low FODMAP Chicken and Vegetable Skewers

Ingredients:
- 1 lb chicken breast, cut into cubes
- 2 zucchinis, sliced
- 1 cup cherry tomatoes
- 2 tablespoons garlic-infused olive oil
- 1 teaspoon dried rosemary
- Salt and pepper to taste

Preparation:
1. Preheat the grill to medium heat.
2. Thread chicken, zucchini, and tomatoes onto skewers.
3. Mix garlic-infused olive oil, rosemary, salt, and pepper. Brush onto skewers.
4. Grill for 10-15 minutes, turning occasionally, until chicken is cooked.

Nutritional Information:
- Calories: 240 per serving
- Protein: 28g
- Fat: 11g
- Carbohydrates: 6g

Eggplant and Tomato Bake

Ingredients:

- 1 large eggplant, sliced
- 2 cups cherry tomatoes, halved
- 1/4 cup fresh basil, chopped
- 2 tablespoons olive oil
- Salt and pepper to taste

Preparation:

1. Preheat the oven to 375°F (190°C).
2. Arrange eggplant slices in a baking dish, top with halved cherry tomatoes and chopped basil.
3. Drizzle with olive oil, sprinkle with salt and pepper.
4. Bake for 25-30 minutes or until the eggplant is tender.

Nutritional Information:

- Calories: 180 per serving
- Protein: 3g
- Fat: 12g
- Carbohydrates: 15g

Spinach and Feta Stuffed Chicken Breast

Ingredients:

- 4 boneless, skinless chicken breasts
- 2 cups fresh spinach, chopped
- 1/2 cup feta cheese, crumbled
- 1 tablespoon olive oil

- 1 teaspoon dried oregano
- Salt and pepper to taste

Preparation:

1. Preheat the oven to 375°F (190°C).

2. Butterfly the chicken breasts and stuff with spinach and feta.

3. Drizzle with olive oil, sprinkle with oregano, salt, and pepper.

4. Bake for 25-30 minutes or until chicken is cooked through.

Nutritional Information:

- Calories: 280 per serving
- Protein: 35g
- Fat: 14g
- Carbohydrates: 3g

Low FODMAP Tofu and Vegetable Stir-Fry

Ingredients:

- 1 block firm tofu, cubed
- 2 cups broccoli florets
- 1 red bell pepper, sliced
- 2 tablespoons low FODMAP stir-fry sauce
- 1 tablespoon sesame oil

Preparation:

1. Press tofu to remove excess water, then stir-fry in sesame oil until golden.

2. Add broccoli and bell pepper, stir-fry until vegetables are tender.

3. Pour in stir-fry sauce, toss, and cook for an additional 2 minutes.

Nutritional Information:

- Calories: 220 per serving
- Protein: 18g
- Fat: 14g
- Carbohydrates: 10g

Low FODMAP Beef and Vegetable Skillet

Ingredients:

- 1 lb lean ground beef
- 2 cups zucchini, sliced
- 1 cup carrots, julienned
- 1 cup green beans, trimmed
- 2 tablespoons tomato paste
- 1 teaspoon dried thyme
- Salt and pepper to taste

Preparation:

1. In a skillet, brown ground beef over medium heat.

2. Add vegetables, tomato paste, thyme, salt, and pepper. Cook until vegetables are tender.

Nutritional Information:

- Calories: 290 per serving
- Protein: 25g

- Fat: 15g
- Carbohydrates: 14g

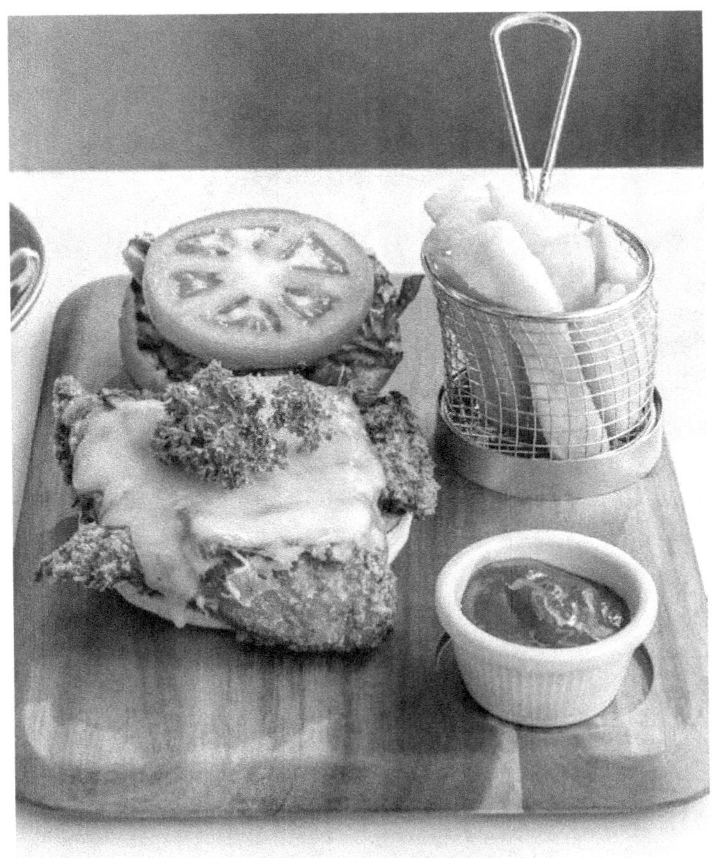

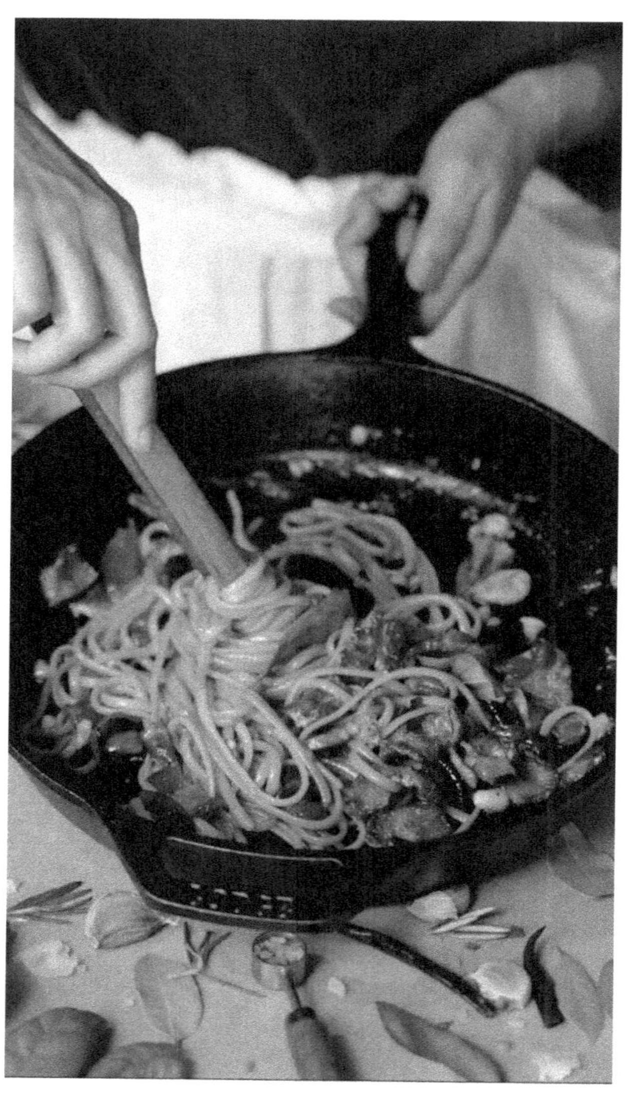

CHAPTER 7:ONE-POT WONDERS

One-Pot Low-FODMAP Chicken and Vegetable Stir Fry

Ingredients:

- 1 pound boneless, skinless chicken breasts, thinly sliced
- 2 tablespoons garlic-infused oil
- 2 cups broccoli florets
- 1 red bell pepper, thinly sliced
- 1 zucchini, sliced into rounds
- 1 cup carrots, julienned
- 1 tablespoon ginger, minced
- 2 tablespoons gluten-free soy sauce
- 1 tablespoon green onion (green parts only), chopped
- 1 tablespoon sesame seeds (optional)
- Salt and pepper to taste

Preparation:

1. In a large skillet or wok, heat the garlic-infused oil over medium-high heat.

2. Add the sliced chicken and cook until browned on all sides.

3. Add ginger to the chicken and stir for about 1 minute.

4. Fill the skillet with broccoli, carrots, zucchini, and red bell pepper. Stir-fry the vegetables for a further five to seven minutes, or until they are crisp-tender.

5. Cover the chicken and veggies with a gluten-free soy sauce. After combining, heat for a further two to three minutes.

6. Season with salt and pepper to taste.

7. Garnish with chopped green onions and sesame seeds if desired.

8. Serve hot and enjoy your delicious one-pot low-FODMAP chicken and vegetable stir fry!

Nutritional Information (per serving, assuming 4 servings):
- Calories: 280
- Protein: 28g
- Carbohydrates: 12g
- Dietary Fiber: 4g
- Sugars: 4g
- Fat: 14g
- Saturated Fat: 2g
- Cholesterol: 73mg
- Sodium: 560mg

One-Pot Low-FODMAP Quinoa and Shrimp Pilaf

Ingredients:
- 1 cup quinoa, rinsed

- 1 pound shrimp, peeled and deveined
- 2 tablespoons olive oil
- 1 red bell pepper, diced
- 1 zucchini, diced
- 1 cup cherry tomatoes, halved
- 1 teaspoon cumin
- 1 teaspoon paprika
- 1 teaspoon dried oregano
- 2 cups low-FODMAP chicken broth
- Salt and pepper to taste
- Fresh parsley, chopped, for garnish

Preparation:

1. Heat the olive oil in a big pot over medium heat. Sauté the zucchini and diced red bell pepper for two to three minutes, or until the vegetables start to soften.

2. Add the shrimp to the stove and simmer for 3–4 minutes, or until they turn pink.

3. Add the dried oregano, cumin, paprika, and quinoa. Simmer for a further two minutes to give the quinoa a chance to lightly roast.

4. Add the low-FODMAP chicken broth to the pot along with the cherry tomatoes.

5. After bringing the mixture to a boil, lower the heat to a simmer, cover it, and cook the quinoa for 15 to 20 minutes, or until it is tender and the liquid has been absorbed.

6. To taste, add salt and pepper for seasoning.

7. Before serving, garnish with freshly cut parsley.

8. Serve hot and enjoy your one-pot low-FODMAP quinoa and shrimp pilaf!

Nutritional Information (per serving, assuming 4 servings):
- Calories: 330
- Protein: 27g
- Carbohydrates: 35g
- Dietary Fiber: 5g
- Sugars: 4g
- Fat: 10g
- Saturated Fat: 1g
- Cholesterol: 160mg
- Sodium: 450mg

One-Pot Low-FODMAP Turkey and Vegetable Chili

Ingredients:
- 1 pound ground turkey
- 1 tablespoon garlic-infused oil
- 1 red bell pepper, diced
- 1 yellow bell pepper, diced
- 1 zucchini, diced
- 1 cup canned diced tomatoes (no onion or garlic added)
- 1 cup canned black beans, drained and rinsed
- 1 cup canned kidney beans, drained and rinsed
- 2 teaspoons ground cumin
- 2 teaspoons paprika

- 1 teaspoon dried oregano
- Half a teaspoon, or according to taste, cayenne pepper
- Two cups chicken broth with low-FODMAPs
- To taste, add salt and pepper.
- Chopped green onions (only the green portions) as a garnish

Preparation:

1. Heat the oil flavored with garlic in a big pot over medium heat. Cook the ground turkey until it turns brown.

2. Add diced red and yellow bell peppers, and zucchini. Sauté for 3-4 minutes until vegetables are slightly softened.

3. Stir in diced tomatoes, black beans, kidney beans, ground cumin, paprika, dried oregano, and cayenne pepper.

4. Pour in low-FODMAP chicken broth and bring the mixture to a simmer.

5. Reduce heat to low, cover, and let it simmer for about 20-25 minutes, allowing flavors to meld.

6. Season with salt and pepper to taste.

7. Garnish with chopped green onions before serving.

8. Serve hot and savor your one-pot low-FODMAP turkey and vegetable chili!

Nutritional Information (per serving, assuming 4 servings):

- Calories: 320
- Protein: 27g

- Carbohydrates: 30g
- Dietary Fiber: 8g
- Sugars: 4g
- Fat: 12g
- Saturated Fat: 2g
- Cholesterol: 60mg
- Sodium: 580mg

One-Pot Low-FODMAP Salmon and Quinoa Skillet

Ingredients:
- 1 cup quinoa, rinsed
- 4 salmon filets
- 2 tablespoons olive oil
- 1 fennel bulb, thinly sliced
- 1 cup cherry tomatoes, halved
- 1 lemon, sliced
- 2 teaspoons dried dill
- 1 teaspoon paprika
- Salt and pepper to taste
- Fresh parsley, chopped, for garnish

Preparation:

1. Heat the olive oil in a big skillet over medium heat. Saute the sliced fennel for three to four minutes, or until it begins to soften.

2. Push the fennel to the sides of the skillet, making space for the salmon filets. Season salmon with paprika, dried dill, salt, and pepper.

3. Place salmon filets in the skillet and sear for 3-4 minutes on each side until golden brown.

4. Add rinsed quinoa to the skillet, arranging it around the salmon.

5. Scatter halved cherry tomatoes and lemon slices over the quinoa and fennel.

6. Pour 2 cups of water over the quinoa and bring the mixture to a simmer.

7. Cover the skillet, reduce heat to low, and let it cook for 15-20 minutes until the quinoa is cooked and the liquid is absorbed.

8. Garnish with fresh parsley before serving.

9. Serve hot and enjoy your one-pot low-FODMAP salmon and quinoa skillet!

Nutritional Information (per serving, assuming 4 servings):

- Calories: 380
- Protein: 32g
- Carbohydrates: 28g
- Dietary Fiber: 5g
- Sugars: 2g
- Fat: 16g
- Saturated Fat: 2.5g
- Cholesterol: 80mg
- Sodium: 220mg

One-Pot Low-FODMAP Beef and Vegetable Stew

Ingredients:

– 1.5 pounds of bite-sized stewing beef chunks

- 2 teaspoons of oil infused with garlic

- Two cups of chopped carrots

- Two cups of green beans, sliced into 2-inch segments

- One cup of sliced celery

- One cup chopped potatoes

- 1 cup chopped parsnips

- A teaspoon of thyme, dried

- Two bay leaves

– Four cups of low-FODMAPS beef stock

To taste, add salt and pepper.

- Chopped fresh chives as a garnish

Preparation:

1. Heat the oil flavored with garlic in a big pot over medium heat. Brown the stewing beef on all sides after adding it.

2. Add carrots, green beans, celery, potatoes, and parsnips to the pot. Stir to combine.

3. Season with dried thyme, bay leaves, salt, and pepper.

4. Pour in the low-FODMAP beef broth and bring the stew to a simmer.

5. Cover the pot and let it simmer for 1.5 to 2 hours or until the beef is tender.

6. Adjust seasoning if needed and remove the bay leaves before serving.

7. Garnish with chopped fresh chives.

8. Serve hot and enjoy your comforting one-pot low-FODMAP beef and vegetable stew!

Nutritional Information (per serving, assuming 4 servings):

- Calories: 400
- Protein: 30g
- Carbohydrates: 30g
- Dietary Fiber: 6g
- Sugars: 4g
- Fat: 18g
- Saturated Fat: 5g
- Cholesterol: 90mg
- Sodium: 800mg

One-Pot Low-FODMAP Shrimp and Quinoa Paella

Ingredients:

- 1 cup quinoa, rinsed
- 1 pound shrimp, peeled and deveined
- 2 tablespoons olive oil
- 1 red bell pepper, diced
- 1 yellow bell pepper, diced
- 1 cup cherry tomatoes, halved
- 1 teaspoon smoked paprika

- 1 teaspoon saffron threads (optional)
- 2 cups low-FODMAP chicken broth
- Salt and pepper to taste
- Fresh cilantro, chopped, for garnish

Preparation:

1. In a large paella pan or skillet, heat olive oil over medium heat. Add diced red and yellow bell peppers and sauté for 3-4 minutes until softened.

2. Add shrimp to the pan and cook until they turn pink, about 3-4 minutes.

3. Stir in quinoa, cherry tomatoes, smoked paprika, and saffron threads.

4. Pour in low-FODMAP chicken broth and bring the mixture to a simmer.

5. Reduce heat to low, cover, and let it simmer for about 20-25 minutes, allowing the quinoa to cook and the liquid to be absorbed.

6. Season with salt and pepper to taste.

7. Garnish with chopped fresh cilantro before serving.

8. Serve hot and savor your one-pot low-FODMAP shrimp and quinoa paella!

Nutritional Information (per serving, assuming 4 servings):

- Calories: 340
- Protein: 28g
- Carbohydrates: 30g
- Dietary Fiber: 5g
- Sugars: 3g

- Fat: 12g
- Saturated Fat: 1.5g
- Cholesterol: 160mg
- Sodium: 450mg

One-Pot Low-FODMAP Eggplant and Chicken Curry

Ingredients:
- 1 pound boneless, skinless chicken thighs, cut into bite-sized pieces
- 2 tablespoons garlic-infused oil
- 1 eggplant, diced
- 1 red bell pepper, sliced
– 1 cup finely chopped 2-inch green beans
- One 14-ounce can of coconut milk
- Two teaspoons of curry powder low in FODMAPS
- One teaspoon of ground turmeric
- One teaspoon of coriander powder
- One teaspoon, or according your taste, cayenne pepper
To taste, add salt and pepper.
- Chopped fresh cilantro as a garnish
- Prepared white rice to serve

Preparation:
1. Heat the oil flavored with garlic over medium heat in a big pot. Cook the chicken until it turns golden brown on all sides.

2. Add diced eggplant, sliced red bell pepper, and green beans to the pot. Stir to combine.

3. In a bowl, mix coconut milk with curry powder, ground turmeric, ground coriander, cayenne pepper, salt, and pepper.

4. Pour the coconut milk mixture over the chicken and vegetables in the pot.

5. Bring the mixture to a simmer, then reduce heat to low, cover, and let it cook for 20-25 minutes or until chicken is cooked through and vegetables are tender.

6. Adjust seasoning if needed.

7. Garnish with chopped fresh cilantro.

8. Serve the curry over cooked white rice and enjoy your one-pot low-FODMAP eggplant and chicken curry!

Nutritional Information (per serving, assuming 4 servings):

- Calories: 420
- Protein: 24g
- Carbohydrates: 20g
- Dietary Fiber: 6g
- Sugars: 6g
- Fat: 30g
- Saturated Fat: 20g
- Cholesterol: 90mg
- Sodium: 380mg

One-Pot Low-FODMAP Lentil and Spinach Soup

Ingredients:
- One cup of rinsed dried green or brown lentils
- 2 tablespoons olive oil
- 1 carrot, diced
- 1 celery stalk, diced
- 1 leek (green parts only), sliced
- 4 cups low-FODMAP vegetable broth
- 1 bay leaf
- 1 teaspoon dried thyme
- 4 cups fresh spinach, chopped
- Salt and pepper to taste
- Lemon wedges for serving

Preparation:
1. Heat the olive oil in a big pot over medium heat. Add the chopped leek, celery, and cubed carrot. The vegetables should soften after 3–4 minutes of sautéing.
2. Add rinsed lentils, low-FODMAP vegetable broth, bay leaf, and dried thyme to the pot. Bring to a boil.
3. Reduce heat to low, cover, and simmer for 20-25 minutes or until lentils are tender.
4. Stir in chopped spinach and cook for an additional 2-3 minutes until the spinach is wilted.
5. Season with salt and pepper to taste.
6. Remove the bay leaf before serving.
7. Serve hot with a wedge of lemon on the side.

8. Enjoy your nutritious one-pot low-FODMAP lentil and spinach soup!

Nutritional Information (per serving, assuming 4 servings):
- Calories: 250
- Protein: 15g
- Carbohydrates: 38g
- Dietary Fiber: 16g
- Sugars: 4g
- Fat: 5g
- Saturated Fat: 0.5g
- Cholesterol: 0mg
- Sodium: 680mg

One-Pot Low-FODMAP Zucchini Noodles with Pesto and Grilled Chicken

Ingredients:
- 1 pound chicken breast, grilled and sliced
- 4 medium-sized zucchini, spiralized into noodles
- 2 tablespoons garlic-infused olive oil
- 1 cup cherry tomatoes, halved
- 1/2 cup pine nuts, toasted
- 1 cup fresh basil leaves
- 1/2 cup grated Parmesan cheese (check for no added garlic or onion)

- 1/2 cup extra virgin olive oil
- Salt and pepper to taste
- Lemon wedges for serving

Preparation:

1. In a food processor, combine fresh basil, grated Parmesan, and toasted pine nuts. Pulse until finely chopped.

2. With the processor running, slowly drizzle in the extra virgin olive oil until a smooth pesto is formed.

3. Heat the garlic-infused olive oil in a large skillet over medium heat. Add zucchini noodles and cherry tomatoes, sautéing for 2-3 minutes until the noodles are just tender.

4. Add the grilled and sliced chicken to the skillet, stirring to combine.

5. Pour the prepared pesto over the zucchini noodles and chicken, tossing to coat evenly.

6. Season with salt and pepper to taste.

7. Serve hot with lemon wedges on the side for a burst of freshness.

Nutritional Information (per serving, assuming 4 servings):

- Calories: 420
- Protein: 32g
- Carbohydrates: 12g
- Dietary Fiber: 4g
- Sugars: 5g
- Fat: 28g

- Saturated Fat: 5g
- Cholesterol: 80mg
- Sodium: 220mg

One-Pot Low-FODMAP Turkey and Quinoa Stuffed Peppers

Ingredients:
- 1 pound ground turkey
- 1 cup quinoa, cooked
- 1 tablespoon garlic-infused olive oil
- 4 bell peppers, halved and seeds removed
- 1 cup tomatoes, diced
- 1 cup zucchini, diced
- 1 cup carrots, grated
- 1 teaspoon ground cumin
- 1 teaspoon smoked paprika
- Salt and pepper to taste
- 1 cup low-FODMAP chicken broth
- Fresh parsley, chopped, for garnish

Preparation:
1. Turn the oven on to 375°F, or 190°C.
2. Heat the olive oil that has been flavored with garlic in a big skillet over medium heat. Cook the ground turkey until it turns brown.
3. Fill the skillet with chopped tomatoes, grated carrots, and zucchini. The vegetables should soften after 3–4 minutes of sautéing.

4. Add the quinoa that has been cooked, smoked paprika, ground cumin, salt, and pepper.

5. Put the bell peppers, cut in half, in a baking dish. Fill each pepper half with a spoonful of the turkey and quinoa mixture.

6. Fill the baking dish with low-FODMAP chicken broth, encircling the peppers.

7. Bake the casserole in a preheated oven for 25 to 30 minutes, or until the peppers are soft, covered with foil.

8. Before serving, garnish with freshly cut parsley.

9. Serve hot and enjoy your one-pot low-FODMAP turkey and quinoa stuffed peppers!

Nutritional Information (per serving, assuming 4 servings):

- Calories: 340
- Protein: 25g
- Carbohydrates: 32g
- Dietary Fiber: 6g
- Sugars: 6g
- Fat: 14g
- Saturated Fat: 2.5g
- Cholesterol: 70mg
- Sodium: 380mg

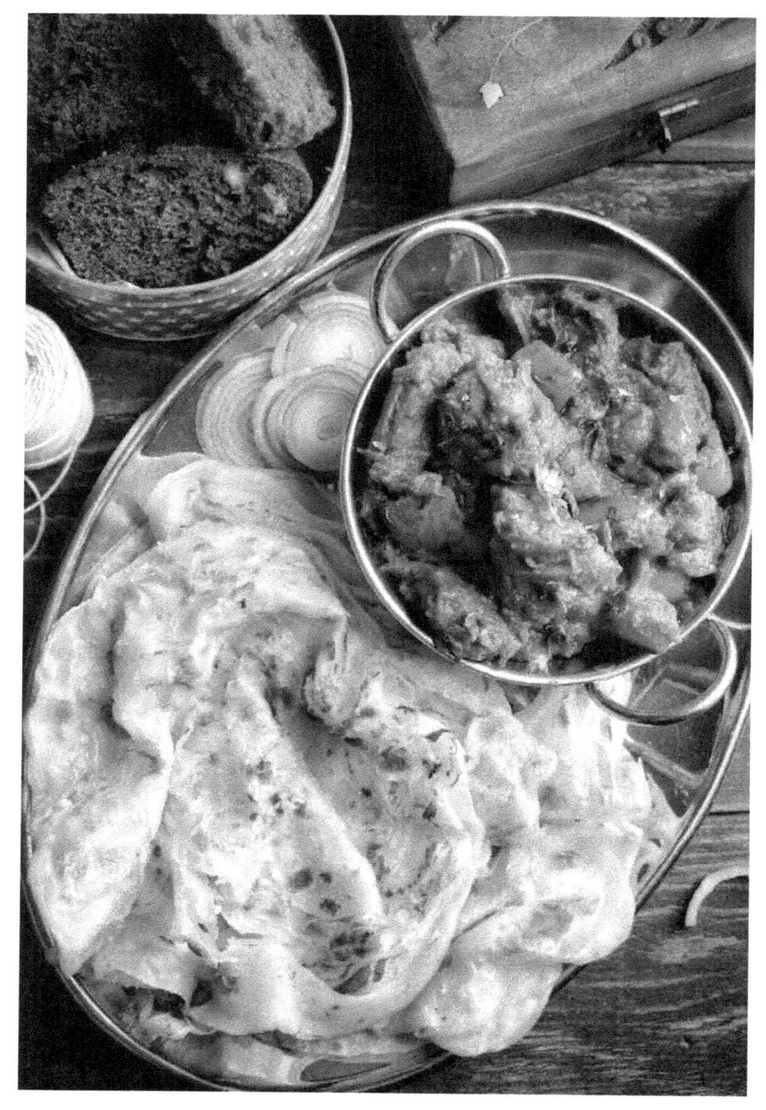

CHAPTER 8: DESSERTS TO SAVOR

Low-FODMAP Banana Almond Muffins:

Ingredients:
- 2 ripe bananas (mashed)
- 1 cup almond flour
- 1/2 cup oat flour
- 1/4 cup maple syrup
- 2 large eggs
- 1/4 cup lactose-free milk
- 1/4 cup coconut oil (melted)
- 1 teaspoon vanilla extract
- 1 teaspoon baking powder
- 1/2 teaspoon baking soda
- 1/4 teaspoon salt
- Optional: 1/3 cup dark chocolate chips (ensure no high-FODMAP ingredients)

Instructions:

1. Grease a muffin tray with paper liners and preheat the oven to 350°F (175°C).

2. Put the mashed bananas, eggs, lactose-free milk, melted coconut oil, almond flour, oat flour, maple syrup, and vanilla extract in a big bowl. Blend thoroughly.

3. Combine the baking soda, baking powder, and salt in another basin. Mix until just mixed, add the dry ingredients to the wet ones.

4. You can optionally mix in dark chocolate chunks.

5. Using a spoon, scoop out the batter and fill each muffin cup about two thirds of the way.

6. Bake the cake for twenty to twenty-five minutes, or until a toothpick inserted in the center comes out clean.

7. Allow the muffins to cool in the tin for 5 minutes before transferring them to a wire rack to cool completely.

Nutritional Information (per muffin):
- Calories: approximately 180
- Protein: 5g
- Fat: 12g
- Carbohydrates: 15g
- Fiber: 2g
- Sugars: 7g

Low-FODMAP Berry Parfait:

Ingredients:
- 1 cup lactose-free Greek yogurt
- One cup of mixed berries like strawberries, blueberries, raspberries
- 2 tablespoons chopped walnuts
- 1 tablespoon chia seeds
- 1 tablespoon maple syrup

Instructions:

1. In a bowl, mix the lactose-free Greek yogurt with maple syrup until well combined.

2. In serving glasses or bowls, layer the yogurt mixture with mixed berries.

3. Sprinkle chopped walnuts and chia seeds on top of each layer.

4. Repeat the layering until the glasses are filled, finishing with a layer of berries, walnuts, and chia seeds on top.

5. Drizzle a little extra maple syrup on the top for sweetness.

6. Refrigerate for at least 30 minutes before serving to allow flavors to meld.

Nutritional Information (per serving):

- Calories: approximately 220

- Protein: 12g

- Fat: 10g

- Carbohydrates: 20g

- Fiber: 6g

- Sugars: 10g

Low-FODMAP Lemon Poppy Seed Cookies:

Ingredients:

- 1 cup almond flour

- 1/4 cup coconut flour

- 1/4 cup melted coconut oil
- 1/4 cup maple syrup
- 1 large egg
- Zest of 1 lemon
- 1 tablespoon lemon juice
- 1 tablespoon poppy seeds
- 1/2 teaspoon baking soda
- 1/4 teaspoon salt

Instructions:

Preheat the oven to 350°F (175°C), and place parchment paper on a baking pan.

2. In a bowl, thoroughly mix the almond flour, coconut flour, egg, lemon zest, lemon juice, poppy seeds, melted coconut oil, maple syrup, baking soda, and salt.

3. Leaving space between each cookie, scoop spoonfuls of dough and set them on the baking sheet that has been prepared.

4. Using your fingertips or the back of a spoon, slightly flatten each cookie.

5. Bake for ten to twelve minutes, or until the sides are browned.

6. Let the cookies cool for a few minutes on the baking sheet, then move them to a wire rack to finish cooling.

Nutritional Information (per cookie):

- Calories: approximately 90
- Protein: 2g
- Fat: 7g
- Carbohydrates: 6g

- Fiber: 1g
- Sugars: 3g

Low-FODMAP Chocolate Avocado Mousse:

Ingredients:
- 2 ripe avocados
- 1/4 cup cocoa powder (ensure no high-FODMAP ingredients)
- 1/4 cup maple syrup
- 1/4 cup lactose-free milk
- 1 teaspoon vanilla extract
- Pinch of salt
- Fresh berries for garnish

Instructions:
1. In a blender or food processor, combine avocados, cocoa powder, maple syrup, lactose-free milk, vanilla extract, and a pinch of salt.
2. Blend, scraping down the sides as necessary, until creamy and smooth.
3. Taste and add additional maple syrup to adjust sweetness if needed.
4. Ladle the mousse of chocolate and avocado into serving cups.
5. To help the mousse firm, place in the refrigerator for at least two hours.
6. Garnish with fresh berries before serving.

Nutritional Information (per serving):
- Calories: approximately 200
- Protein: 3g
- Fat: 14g
- Carbohydrates: 21g
- Fiber: 7g
- Sugars: 11g

Low-FODMAP Pumpkin Spice Energy Bites:

Ingredients:
- 1 cup canned pumpkin puree (check for no added high-FODMAP ingredients)
- 1 cup rolled oats
- 1/4 cup chia seeds
- 1/4 cup maple syrup
- 1/2 cup shredded coconut (unsweetened)
- 1 teaspoon pumpkin spice blend
- 1/4 cup chopped pecans (optional)

Instructions:
1. In a large bowl, combine the pumpkin puree, rolled oats, chia seeds, maple syrup, shredded coconut, pumpkin spice blend, and chopped pecans (if using).
2. Mix the ingredients until well combined.
3. Place the bowl in the refrigerator for about 30 minutes to allow the mixture to firm up.

4. After chilling, roll the mixture into bite-sized balls using your hands.

5. Store the energy bites in an airtight container in the refrigerator.

Nutritional Information (per energy bite):

- Calories: approximately 70
- Protein: 2g
- Fat: 3g
- Carbohydrates: 10g
- Fiber: 2g
- Sugars: 3g

Low-FODMAP Mint Chocolate Chip Smoothie:

Ingredients:

- 1 cup lactose-free milk (e.g., almond, coconut, or lactose-free cow's milk)
- 1 cup fresh spinach leaves
- 1/2 banana (ripe, peeled)
- 1/4 teaspoon peppermint extract
- 1 tablespoon dark chocolate chips (ensure no high-FODMAP ingredients)
- Ice cubes (optional)

Instructions:

1. In a blender, combine lactose-free milk, fresh spinach leaves, banana, and peppermint extract.

2. Blend until smooth and creamy.

3. Add dark chocolate chips to the blender and pulse a few times to incorporate.

4. If desired, add ice cubes and blend again until the smoothie reaches your preferred consistency.

5. Pour the mint chocolate chip smoothie into a glass and enjoy immediately.

Nutritional Information:

- Calories: approximately 150
- Protein: 4g
- Fat: 7g
- Carbohydrates: 18g
- Fiber: 3g
- Sugars: 9g

Low-FODMAP Cinnamon Pecan Rice Pudding:

Ingredients:

- 1 cup cooked white rice (cooled)
- 1 1/2 cups lactose-free milk
- 1/4 cup maple syrup
- 1 teaspoon ground cinnamon
- 1/4 cup chopped pecans
- 1 teaspoon vanilla extract
- Pinch of salt

Instructions:

1. In a saucepan, combine the cooked rice, lactose-free milk, maple syrup, ground cinnamon, and a pinch of salt.

2. Cook over medium heat, stirring frequently, until the mixture thickens and the rice absorbs the flavors (about 15-20 minutes).

3. Once the rice pudding has thickened, remove it from heat and stir in the chopped pecans and vanilla extract.

4. Allow the rice pudding to cool before serving.

5. Optionally, sprinkle a bit of extra cinnamon on top for garnish.

Nutritional Information (per serving):

- Calories: approximately 220
- Protein: 5g
- Fat: 7g
- Carbohydrates: 35g
- Fiber: 2g
- Sugars: 14g

Low-FODMAP Raspberry Coconut Chia Pudding:

Ingredients:

- 1/4 cup chia seeds
- 1 cup lactose-free coconut milk
- 1 tablespoon maple syrup
- 1/2 teaspoon vanilla extract
- 1/2 cup fresh raspberries
- 2 tablespoons shredded coconut (unsweetened)

Instructions:

1. In a bowl, mix chia seeds, lactose-free coconut milk, maple syrup, and vanilla extract.

2. Stir well and let the mixture sit for 5 minutes.

3. After 5 minutes, stir the mixture again to prevent clumping, then cover and refrigerate for at least 2 hours or overnight.

4. Once the chia pudding has set, layer it in serving glasses with fresh raspberries.

5. Top each layer with a sprinkle of shredded coconut.

6. Serve chilled and enjoy!

Nutritional Information (per serving):

- Calories: approximately 180
- Protein: 4g
- Fat: 10g
- Carbohydrates: 20g
- Fiber: 10g
- Sugars: 6g

Low-FODMAP Almond Butter Banana Bites:

Ingredients:

- 2 bananas (ripe but firm)
- 2 tablespoons almond butter
- 2 tablespoons chopped almonds
- 1 tablespoon chia seeds
- 1/2 teaspoon cinnamon

Instructions:

1. Peel the bananas and cut them into bite-sized rounds.

2. Spread a small amount of almond butter on each banana round.

3. In a shallow dish, combine chopped almonds, chia seeds, and cinnamon.

4. Dip each almond butter-coated banana round into the almond, chia, and cinnamon mixture, coating all sides.

5. Place the coated banana bites on a plate or tray lined with parchment paper.

6. Refrigerate for at least 30 minutes to allow the bites to firm up before serving.

Nutritional Information (per serving):

- Calories: approximately 120
- Protein: 3g
- Fat: 7g
- Carbohydrates: 13g
- Fiber: 3g
- Sugars: 6g

Low-FODMAP Blueberry Oatmeal Muffins:

Ingredients:

- 1 cup rolled oats
- 1 cup oat flour
- 1/2 cup lactose-free milk
- 1/4 cup maple syrup

- 1/4 cup coconut oil (melted)
- 2 teaspoons baking powder
- 1/2 teaspoon cinnamon
- 1/4 teaspoon salt
- 1 cup fresh blueberries

Instructions:

1. Grease a muffin tray with paper liners and preheat the oven to 350°F (175°C).

2. Combine the rolled oats, oat flour, baking powder, cinnamon, and salt in a big basin.

3. Combine the melted coconut oil, maple syrup, and lactose-free milk in a another bowl.

4. Combine the wet and dry ingredients, stirring just until blended.

5. Fold in the fresh blueberries gently.

6. Using a spoon, scoop out the batter and fill each muffin cup about two thirds of the way.

7. Bake for 18 to 20 minutes, or until an inserted toothpick comes out clean.

8. After the muffins have cooled in the pan for five minutes, move them to a wire rack to finish cooling.

Nutritional Information (per muffin):

- Calories: approximately 150
- Protein: 3g
- Fat: 7g
- Carbohydrates: 18g
- Fiber: 2g
- Sugars: 6g

CHAPTER 9: BEVERAGES FOR EVERY OCCASION

Minty Green Tea Cooler

Ingredients:
- 2 green tea bags
- 1 tablespoon fresh mint leaves, chopped
- 1 tablespoon maple syrup (ensure it's 100% pure maple syrup)
- 1/2 lime, juiced
- Ice cubes

Preparation:
1. Boil 2 cups of water and steep the green tea bags for 3-4 minutes.
2. When the tea reaches room temperature, remove the tea bags and let it cool.
3. In a blender, combine the cooled green tea, chopped mint leaves, maple syrup, and lime juice. Blend until smooth.
4. Strain the mixture to remove 9 mint leaves.
5. Pour the mixture over ice cubes in a glass and garnish with a mint sprig.
6. Enjoy your refreshing Minty Green Tea Cooler!

Nutritional Information (per serving):
- Calories: 30 kcal
- Protein: 0.5g
- Fat: 0g
- Carbohydrates: 7g
- Fiber: 0.5g

Berry Citrus Sparkler

Ingredients:
- One cup of mixed berries (strawberries, blueberries, raspberries)
- 1 orange, juiced
- 1 tablespoon honey
- 2 cups sparkling water
- Ice cubes

Preparation:
1. In a blender, combine the mixed berries, orange juice, and honey. Blend until smooth.
2. Strain the mixture to get rid of the pulp and seeds.
3. Fill glasses with ice cubes and pour the berry-orange mixture evenly among them.
4. Top each glass with sparkling water and gently stir.
5. Garnish with a slice of orange or a few whole berries.
6. Sip and savor your delightful Berry Citrus Sparkler!

Nutritional Information (per serving):
- Calories: 50 kcal
- Protein: 0.5g

- Fat: 0g
- Carbohydrates: 12g
- Fiber: 2.5g

Cucumber Mint Infused Water

Ingredients:
- 1/2 cucumber, thinly sliced
- 1/4 cup fresh mint leaves
- 1 lemon, thinly sliced
- 1 teaspoon grated ginger (optional)
- 4 cups water
- Ice cubes

Preparation:
1. In a large pitcher, combine cucumber slices, mint leaves, lemon slices, and grated ginger.
2. Pour water over the ingredients and refrigerate for at least 2 hours to allow flavors to infuse.
3. Serve over ice and garnish with a sprig of mint or a cucumber wheel.
4. Enjoy the refreshing taste of Cucumber Mint Infused Water!

Nutritional Information (per serving):
- Calories: 5 kcal
- Protein: 0g
- Fat: 0g
- Carbohydrates: 1g
- Fiber: 0.5g

Pineapple Coconut Smoothie

Ingredients:

- 1 cup fresh pineapple, diced
- 1/2 cup coconut milk (check for no added high-FODMAP ingredients)
- 1/2 cup lactose-free yogurt
- 1 tablespoon chia seeds
- 1 teaspoon vanilla extract
- Ice cubes

Preparation:

1. In a blender, combine fresh pineapple, coconut milk, lactose-free yogurt, chia seeds, and vanilla extract.

2. Blend until smooth and creamy.

3. Add ice cubes and blend again until the smoothie reaches your desired consistency.

4. Pour into a glass and enjoy the tropical flavors of Pineapple Coconut Smoothie!

Nutritional Information (per serving):

- Calories: 200 kcal
- Protein: 3g
- Fat: 11g
- Carbohydrates: 24g
- Fiber: 5g

Iced Peppermint Chamomile Tea

Ingredients:
- 2 peppermint tea bags
- 2 chamomile tea bags
- 1 tablespoon maple syrup (optional)
- 1 lemon, sliced
- Fresh mint leaves for garnish
- Ice cubes

Preparation:

1. Boil 4 cups of water and steep the peppermint and chamomile tea bags for about 5 minutes.

2. Take out the tea bags and allow the tea to cool until it reaches room temperature.

3. Stir in maple syrup if desired.

4. Refrigerate the tea until chilled.

5. Fill glasses with ice cubes and pour the chilled tea over the ice.

6. Garnish with lemon slices and fresh mint leaves.

7. Stir and enjoy the soothing Iced Peppermint Chamomile Tea!

Nutritional Information (per serving):
- Calories: 10 kcal
- Protein: 0g
- Fat: 0g
- Carbohydrates: 2g
- Fiber: 0.5g

Raspberry Lemonade Sparkler

Ingredients:

- 1 cup fresh raspberries
- 1/4 cup freshly squeezed lemon juice
- 2 tablespoons maple syrup (ensure it's 100% pure)
- 2 cups sparkling water
- Lemon slices for garnish
- Ice cubes

Preparation:

1. In a blender, puree the fresh raspberries until smooth.
2. Strain the raspberry puree to remove seeds.
3. In a pitcher, combine the raspberry puree, freshly squeezed lemon juice, and maple syrup.
4. Stir until well mixed.
5. Fill glasses with ice cubes and pour the raspberry-lemon mixture over the ice.
6. Top each glass with sparkling water.
7. Garnish with lemon slices.
8. Sip and enjoy the delightful Raspberry Lemonade Sparkler!

Nutritional Information (per serving):

- Calories: 70 kcal
- Protein: 0.5g
- Fat: 0g
- Carbohydrates: 18g
- Fiber: 3g

Turmeric Ginger Golden Milk

Ingredients:

- 1 cup unsweetened almond milk
- 1/2 teaspoon ground turmeric
- 1/2 teaspoon ground ginger
- 1 tablespoon maple syrup (optional)
- 1/4 teaspoon ground cinnamon
- Pinch of black pepper (helps enhance turmeric absorption)
- Ice cubes

Preparation:

1. Heat the almond milk in a small saucepan over medium heat, being careful not to boil.
2. Whisk in the turmeric, ginger, maple syrup (if using), cinnamon, and black pepper.
3. Continue to heat and whisk until well combined and heated through.
4. Allow the mixture to cool slightly.
5. Pour over ice cubes in a glass.
6. Stir and enjoy the anti-inflammatory goodness of Turmeric Ginger Golden Milk!

Nutritional Information (per serving):

- Calories: 40 kcal
- Protein: 1g
- Fat: 2g
- Carbohydrates: 5g
- Fiber: 1g

Citrus Berry Spritzer

Ingredients:

- One cup of mixed berries, comprising raspberries, blueberries, and strawberries
- One juiced orange
- Juiced one lime
- Two tsp pure maple syrup
- Two cups of Coke
- Cubes of ice

Preparation:

1. Place mixed berries, orange juice, lime juice, and maple syrup in a blender. Process till smooth.
2. Strain the mixture to get rid of the pulp and seeds.
3. Fill glasses with ice cubes and pour the berry-citrus mixture over the ice.
4. Top each glass with club soda.
5. Gently stir and garnish with a slice of orange or lime.
6. Enjoy the fizzy and fruity goodness of Citrus Berry Spritzer!

Nutritional Information (per serving):

- Calories: 60 kcal
- Protein: 0.5g
- Fat: 0g
- Carbohydrates: 15g
- Fiber: 2.5g

CHAPTER 10: MEAL PREP AND PLANNING

Batch Cooking for Convenience

Batch cooking is a fantastic strategy for convenience, especially when following a low-FODMAP (Fermentable Oligosaccharides, Disaccharides, Monosaccharides, and Polyols) diet. This diet is often recommended for individuals with irritable bowel syndrome (IBS) or other gastrointestinal issues. **Here's a guide on low-FODMAP batch cooking for convenience:**
Planning:

1. Create a Meal Plan:
   - Plan your meals for the week, ensuring they adhere to low-FODMAP guidelines.
   - Consider variety to avoid monotony and ensure you get a range of nutrients.
2. Choose Recipes:
   - Opt for recipes that can be easily scaled up and freeze well.
   - Examples include soups, stews, casseroles, and stir-fries.

Shopping:

3. Make a Shopping List:

- Make an extensive shopping list based on your meal plan.

Verify compliance by looking up each item's FODMAP content.

4. Buy in Bulk:

- To save money, buy non-perishable goods in large quantities.

  - Keep them somewhere dry and cool.

Batch Cooking:

5. Purchase Storage Containers:

- Keep a range of containers on hand for freezing and cooling food.

  - Write the contents and the date on them.

6. Batch Cook Proteins:

  - Cook a large batch of low-FODMAP proteins like chicken, turkey, or firm tofu.

  - Season them with permitted herbs and spices.

7. Prepare Low-FODMAP Grains:

  - Cook a batch of quinoa, rice, or other low-FODMAP grains.

  - Portion them into containers for easy access.

8.Make Low-FODMAP Sauces and Dressings:

  - Prepare sauces and dressings in large quantities using low-FODMAP ingredients.

  - Store them separately to add variety to your meals.

9. Cook Vegetables:

   - Choose low-FODMAP vegetables like carrots, zucchini, and bell peppers.

   - Roast or steam them in bulk.

10. Create One-Pot Meals:

   - Prepare soups, stews, or casseroles with a mix of proteins, grains, and vegetables.

   - Divide into portions for freezing.

Storage:

11. Freeze Individual Portions:

   - Portion out meals into individual containers for easy thawing and reheating.

   - Freeze them flat for efficient storage.

12. Make All Labels:

   - Make sure that containers are clearly labeled with preparation date and reheating instructions.

   - Label items with color codes to make identification simple.

Meal Preparation:

13. Thawing and Reheating:

   - Plan ahead and transfer frozen meals to the refrigerator the night before.

   - Reheat in the microwave or on the stove, adding fresh herbs for flavor.

14. Add Fresh Elements:

   - Incorporate fresh low-FODMAP ingredients like herbs, greens, or a squeeze of lemon to enhance flavors.

15. Maintain Variety:
    - Rotate through your frozen meals to maintain a varied and balanced diet.

Batch cooking is an excellent time-saving strategy, and with careful planning, it can be adapted to fit the requirements of a low-FODMAP diet.

Weekly Low FODMAP Meal Planner

The Low FODMAP diet is designed to help people with irritable bowel syndrome (IBS) by restricting certain types of carbohydrates that can trigger digestive symptoms. Here's a sample weekly Low FODMAP meal planner for you. Keep in mind that individual tolerance to specific foods can vary, so it's essential to tailor the plan to your specific needs and preferences.

Day 1:

Breakfast:
- Scrambled eggs with spinach and cherry tomatoes
- Gluten-free toast
Lunch:
- Grilled chicken salad with mixed greens, cucumber, and carrots

- Quinoa
Dinner:
- Baked salmon
- Roasted sweet potatoes
- Steamed green beans
Snack:
- FODMAP-friendly fruit (e.g., strawberries, blueberries)

Day 2:

Breakfast:
- Greek yogurt with a handful of raspberries
- Low FODMAP granola
Lunch:
- Turkey and lettuce wrap with gluten-free tortilla
- Sliced cucumber and carrot sticks with hummus
Dinner:
- Stir-fried tofu with broccoli, bell peppers, and zucchini
- Brown rice
Snack:
- Rice cakes with lactose-free cheese

Day 3:

Breakfast:
- Smoothie with banana (unripe), spinach, lactose-free yogurt, and ice

Lunch:
- Quinoa salad with cucumber, feta cheese, and cherry tomatoes
Dinner:
- Grilled shrimp skewers
- Mashed potatoes made with lactose-free milk
Snack:
- Nuts (almonds, walnuts, or macadamia nuts)

Day 4:

Breakfast:
- Omelet with bell peppers, cheddar cheese, and chives
- Gluten-free toast
Lunch:
- Spinach and feta stuffed chicken breast
- Steamed asparagus
Dinner:
- Low FODMAP spaghetti with homemade tomato sauce (without onion and garlic)
- Grated Parmesan cheese
Snack:
- Carrot and cucumber sticks with a side of low FODMAP dip

Day 5:

Breakfast:
- Lactose-free yogurt parfait with strawberries and a sprinkle of granola
Lunch:
- Quinoa bowl with grilled chicken, cherry tomatoes, and arugula
- Lemon vinaigrette dressing
Dinner:
- Baked cod with lemon and herbs
- Quinoa pilaf with mixed vegetables
Snack:
- Hard-boiled eggs

Day 6:

Breakfast:
- Overnight oats made with gluten-free oats, lactose-free yogurt, and a handful of blueberries
Lunch:
- Turkey and cranberry sauce sandwich on gluten-free bread
- Mixed green salad with a simple olive oil and vinegar dressing
Dinner:

- Grilled steak with rosemary and garlic-infused oil (ensure the garlic is removed)
- Roasted carrots and parsnips
Snack:
- FODMAP-friendly fruit smoothie (e.g., kiwi, pineapple, and strawberries)

Day 7:

Breakfast:
- Banana (unripe) and almond butter smoothie
- Gluten-free toast with lactose-free cream cheese
Lunch:
- Quinoa and spinach-stuffed bell peppers
- Side of sliced cucumbers with a sprinkle of salt
Dinner:
- Chicken stir-fry with bok choy, carrots, and bamboo shoots
- Jasmine rice
Snack:
- Popcorn (plain, without added high FODMAP flavorings)

Remember to stay hydrated throughout the day and adjust portion sizes based on your individual needs. It's also crucial to listen to your body and note any reactions to specific foods.

Tips for Successful Low FODMAP Meal Prep

Following a low FODMAP diet can be challenging, but with careful planning and preparation, it becomes more manageable. Here are some tips for successful low FODMAP meal prep:

1. Educate Yourself: Familiarize yourself with the low FODMAP food list. Understand which foods are high and low in FODMAPs so that you can make informed choices during meal prep.

2. Prepare Your Meals: Make a weekly food plan in advance. This guarantees that you have all the ingredients you need on hand and assists you in making a shopping list.

3. Variety is Key: Ensure your meals are varied to prevent boredom and ensure you're getting a range of nutrients. Rotate your protein sources, include a variety of vegetables, and experiment with different herbs and spices to add flavor.

4. Batch Cooking: Prepare larger quantities of low FODMAP meals and freeze them in individual portions. This makes it convenient for days when you don't have time to cook.

5. Stock Up on Low FODMAP Staples: Keep your pantry stocked with low FODMAP staples like rice, quinoa, gluten-free oats, canned tomatoes, and canned tuna. These items can be the base for many low FODMAP meals.

6. Pre-cut Vegetables and Fruits: Save time by pre-cutting low FODMAP vegetables and fruits. Store them in portion-sized containers in the fridge for easy access.

7. Use Garlic and Onion Alternatives: Since garlic and onions are high in FODMAPs, use their low FODMAP alternatives like garlic-infused oil or green parts of spring onions (scallions) to add flavor to your dishes.

8. Experiment with Herbs and Spices: Enhance the flavor of your dishes with low FODMAP herbs and spices. Common options include basil, oregano, thyme, rosemary, and ginger.

9. Mindful Portioning: Be mindful of portion sizes to avoid consuming excessive FODMAPs unintentionally. Pay attention to the recommended serving sizes for various foods.

10. Keep a Food Diary: Record your meals and any symptoms you experience. This can help you identify trigger foods and tailor your low FODMAP diet more effectively.

11. Read Labels: Always read food labels to check for hidden FODMAPs in processed foods. Look out for ingredients like high fructose corn syrup, inulin, and certain sugar alcohols.

12. Stay Hydrated: Drink plenty of water throughout the day. Proper hydration is essential for overall well-being and can help with digestion.

13. Consult a Dietitian: If you're struggling with the low FODMAP diet or have specific dietary needs, consider consulting a registered dietitian with expertise in the low FODMAP approach.

Remember, the low FODMAP diet is often used as a short-term elimination phase to identify trigger foods.

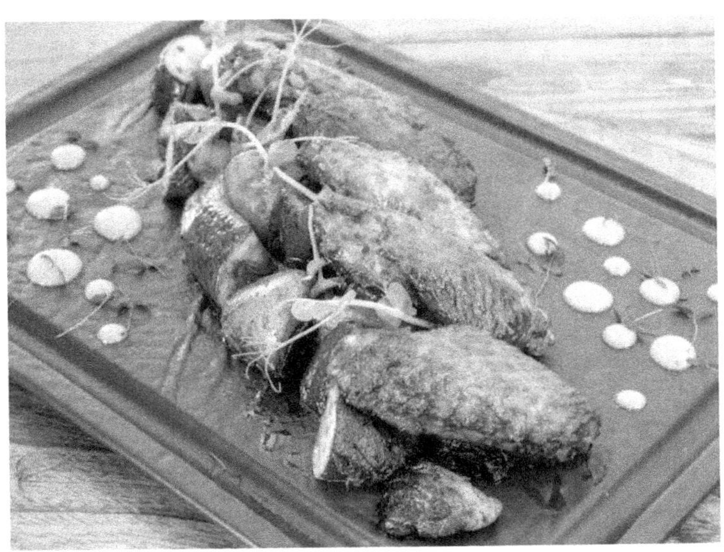

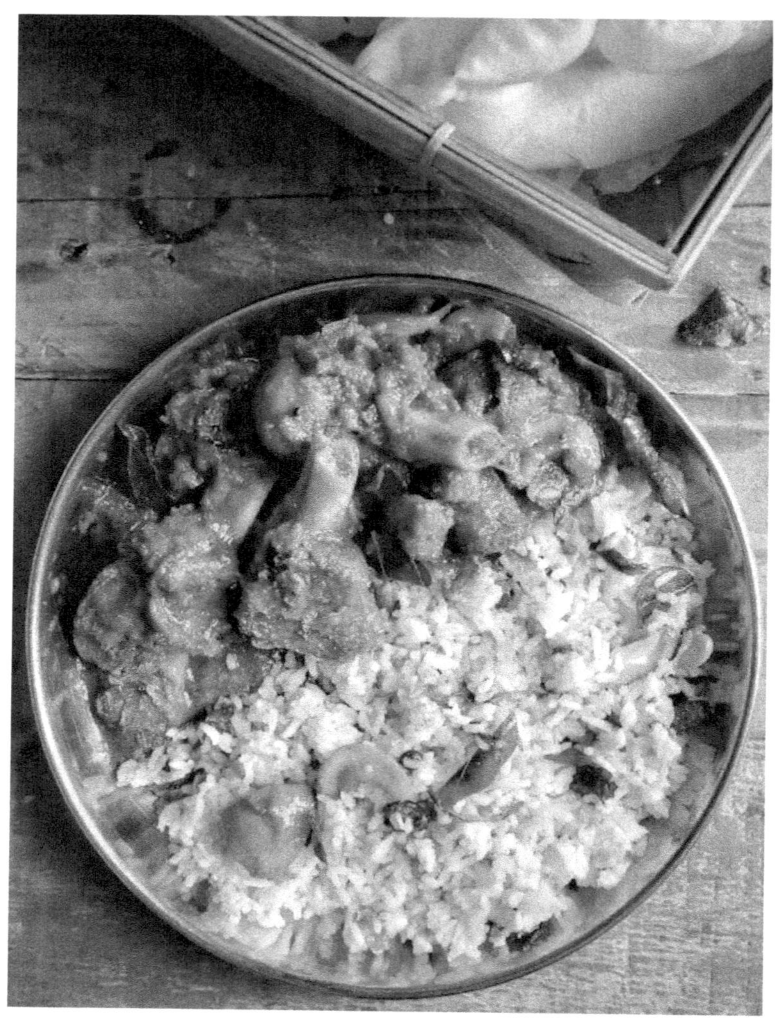

CHAPTER 11: SPECIAL OCCASION RECIPES

Low FODMAP Holiday Roast

Low FODMAP Herb-Roasted Turkey

Ingredients:
- 1 whole turkey (12-14 pounds)
- 1/2 cup garlic-infused olive oil
- 2 tablespoons fresh rosemary, chopped
- 2 tablespoons fresh thyme, chopped
- 2 tablespoons fresh sage, chopped
- Salt and pepper to taste
- 1 lemon, sliced
- 1 cup low FODMAP chicken broth

Preparation:
1. Preheat your oven to 325°F (163°C).
2. Use paper towels to pat dry after rinsing the turkey.
3. In a small bowl, mix the garlic-infused olive oil, chopped rosemary, thyme, sage, salt, and pepper to create a herb-infused oil.

4. Carefully loosen the skin of the turkey, and rub the herb-infused oil under the skin and all over the turkey.

5. Place the lemon slices inside the turkey cavity.

6. Tie the turkey legs together with kitchen twine, and place the turkey on a roasting rack in a roasting pan.

7. Pour the low FODMAP chicken broth into the bottom of the pan.

8. Roast the turkey in the preheated oven, basting occasionally with the pan juices, until the internal temperature reaches 165°F (74°C) in the thickest part of the thigh.

9. Allow the turkey to rest for 20 minutes before carving.

Nutritional Information:

Note: Nutritional values can vary based on the size of the turkey and specific ingredients used.

- Calories: Approximately 350 calories per 4-ounce (113 grams) serving
- Protein: 25g
- Fat: 20g
- Carbohydrates: 0g
- Fiber: 0g
- Sugars: 0g

Low FODMAP Herb-Crusted Beef Tenderloin

Ingredients:

- 1 whole beef tenderloin (4-5 pounds)

- 2 tablespoons olive oil
- 2 tablespoons fresh thyme, chopped
- 2 tablespoons fresh rosemary, chopped
- 2 tablespoons fresh parsley, chopped
- Salt and pepper to taste

Preparation:

1. Preheat your oven to 425°F (218°C).

2. Trim excess fat from the beef tenderloin and tie it with kitchen twine if needed.

3. In a small bowl, mix olive oil, chopped thyme, rosemary, parsley, salt, and pepper to create a herb crust.

4. Rub the herb crust mixture all over the beef tenderloin.

5. Place the beef tenderloin on a rack in a roasting pan.

6. Roast in the preheated oven for about 30-40 minutes or until the internal temperature reaches your desired level of doneness (e.g., 135°F/57°C for medium-rare).

7. Allow the beef tenderloin to rest for 15 minutes before slicing.

Nutritional Information:

Note: Nutritional values can vary based on the size of the beef tenderloin and specific ingredients used.*

- Calories: Approximately 400 calories per 4-ounce (113 grams) serving
- Protein: 30g
- Fat: 30g
- Carbohydrates: 0g
- Fiber: 0g

- Sugars: 0g

Low FODMAP Maple Glazed Ham

Ingredients:
- 1 bone-in ham (7-9 pounds), fully cooked
- 1/2 cup pure maple syrup
- 2 tablespoons Dijon mustard
- 1 tablespoon olive oil
- 1 teaspoon ground cinnamon
- 1/2 teaspoon ground ginger
- 1/4 teaspoon ground cloves

Preparation:
1. Preheat your oven to 325°F (163°C).
2. Put the ham in a roasting pan on a rack.
3. In a small bowl, whisk together maple syrup, Dijon mustard, olive oil, cinnamon, ginger, and cloves to create the glaze.
4. Brush the ham with the maple glaze, making sure to get it into any scored portions of the ham.
5. Tent the ham with aluminum foil and bake in the preheated oven, basting with the glaze every 30 minutes.
6. Bake until the internal temperature reaches 140°F (60°C), uncovering the ham for the last 15-20 minutes to allow the glaze to caramelize.
7. Allow the ham to rest for 15 minutes before slicing.

Nutritional Information:

Note: Nutritional values can vary based on the size of the ham and specific ingredients used.

- Calories: Approximately 250 calories per 4-ounce (113 grams) serving
- Protein: 25g
- Fat: 15g
- Carbohydrates: 5g
- Fiber: 0g
- Sugars: 5g

Low FODMAP Herb-Roasted Chicken

Ingredients:

- 1 whole chicken (about 4 pounds)
- 1/4 cup garlic-infused olive oil
- 2 tablespoons fresh thyme, chopped
- 2 tablespoons fresh rosemary, chopped
- Salt and pepper to taste
- 1 lemon, halved
- 1 cup low FODMAP chicken broth

Preparation:

1. Preheat your oven to 375°F (190°C).
2. Use paper towels to pat the chicken dry after rinsing it.
3. In a small bowl, mix the garlic-infused olive oil, chopped thyme, rosemary, salt, and pepper.

4. Rub the herb-infused oil all over the chicken, including under the skin.

5. Place the lemon halves inside the chicken cavity.

6. Tie the chicken legs together with kitchen twine and place it on a rack in a roasting pan.

7. Pour the low FODMAP chicken broth into the bottom of the pan.

8. Roast the chicken in the preheated oven, basting occasionally, until the internal temperature reaches 165°F (74°C) in the thickest part of the thigh.

9. Allow the chicken to rest for 15 minutes before carving.

Nutritional Information:

Note: Nutritional values can vary based on the size of the chicken and specific ingredients used.

- Calories: Approximately 300 calories per 4-ounce (113 grams) serving
- Protein: 25g
- Fat: 20g
- Carbohydrates: 0g
- Fiber: 0g
- Sugars: 0g

Low FODMAP Cranberry Glazed Pork Tenderloin

Ingredients:

- Two pork tenderloins (about 1.5 pounds each)

- 1 cup fresh cranberries
- 1/2 cup pure maple syrup
- 2 tablespoons balsamic vinegar
- 1 teaspoon Dijon mustard
- 1 tablespoon olive oil
- Salt and pepper to taste
- Fresh rosemary for garnish (optional)

Preparation:

1. Preheat your oven to 375°F (190°C).

2. Use salt and pepper to season the pork tenderloins.

3. Put the cranberries, olive oil, balsamic vinegar, Dijon mustard, and maple syrup in a saucepan. Simmer on medium heat until the sauce thickens and the cranberries pop.

4. Place the pork tenderloins in a roasting pan and brush them with the cranberry glaze.

5. Roast in the preheated oven for about 25-30 minutes or until the internal temperature reaches 145°F (63°C).

6. Let the pork tenderloins rest for 10 minutes before slicing.

7. Garnish with fresh rosemary if desired and serve with additional cranberry glaze on the side.

Nutritional Information:

Note: Nutritional values can vary based on the size of the pork tenderloins and specific ingredients used.

- Calories: Approximately 250 calories per 4-ounce (113 grams) serving
- Protein: 25g

- Fat: 8g
- Carbohydrates: 20g
- Fiber: 2g
- Sugars: 15g

Low FODMAP Lemon Herb Salmon

Ingredients:
- 4 salmon filets (6 ounces each)
- 2 tablespoons fresh dill, chopped
- 2 tablespoons fresh parsley, chopped
- Zest of 1 lemon
- 2 tablespoons olive oil
- Salt and pepper to taste
- Lemon wedges for serving

Preparation:
1. Preheat your oven to 400°F (204°C).
2. In a small bowl, mix together the chopped dill, parsley, lemon zest, olive oil, salt, and pepper.
3. Arrange the salmon filets on a parchment paper-lined baking sheet.
4. Drizzle each salmon filet with the herb and lemon mixture.
5. Bake for 12 to 15 minutes, or until a fork can easily pierce the salmon, in a preheated oven.
6. Present the salmon accompanied by wedges of lemon.

Nutritional Information:

Note: Nutritional values can vary based on the size of the salmon filets and specific ingredients used.*

- Calories: Approximately 300 calories per 6-ounce (170 grams) serving
- Protein: 35g
- Fat: 16g
- Carbohydrates: 1g
- Fiber: 0g
- Sugars: 0g

Mocktail Recipes for Festive Gatherings

Berry Citrus Sparkler

Ingredients:
- 1 cup fresh strawberries, hulled
- 1 cup fresh blueberries
- 1 cup fresh raspberries
- 2 cups cold water
- 1 tablespoon maple syrup
- 1 tablespoon freshly squeezed lime juice
- 2 cups sparkling water
- Ice cubes
- Mint leaves for garnish

Preparation:

1. In a blender, combine strawberries, blueberries, raspberries, cold water, maple syrup, and lime juice.

2. Blend until smooth.

3. Strain the mixture to remove seeds and pulp, obtaining a smooth berry mixture.

4. Fill serving glasses with ice cubes.

5. Pour the berry mixture equally into each glass.

6. Top each glass with sparkling water and gently stir to combine.

7. Garnish with mint leaves.

8. Serve immediately and enjoy your refreshing Berry Citrus Sparkler!

Nutritional Information:

- Serving Size: 1 glass
- Calories: 50 kcal
- Total Fat: 0.3g
- Saturated Fat: 0g
- Cholesterol: 0mg
- Sodium: 8mg
- Total Carbohydrates: 12g
- Dietary Fiber: 3g
- Sugars: 6g
- Protein: 1g

Cucumber Mint Cooler

Ingredients:
- 2 medium-sized cucumbers, peeled and sliced
- 1/4 cup fresh mint leaves
- 1 tablespoon fresh lime juice
- 1 tablespoon maple syrup
- 2 cups cold water
- 2 cups cucumber-flavored sparkling water
- Ice cubes
- Use cucumber slices and mint sprigs for garnish

Preparation:
1. In a blender, combine cucumber slices, mint leaves, lime juice, and maple syrup.
2. Blend until smooth.
3. Strain the cucumber-mint mixture to remove any solids.
4. Fill serving glasses with ice cubes.
5. Pour the cucumber-mint mixture equally into each glass.
6. Top each glass with cold water and cucumber-flavored sparkling water, adjusting to your taste preference.
7. Stir gently to combine.
8. Garnish with cucumber slices and mint sprigs.
9. Serve immediately and savor the coolness of your Cucumber Mint Cooler!

Nutritional Information:
- Serving Size: 1 glass
- Calories: 30 kcal
- Total Fat: 0.1g
- Saturated Fat: 0g
- Cholesterol: 0mg
- Sodium: 7mg
- Total Carbohydrates: 7g
- Dietary Fiber: 1g
- Sugars: 4g
- Protein: 0.5g

Tropical Ginger Zinger

Ingredients:
- 1 cup pineapple chunks (fresh or canned in natural juice)
- 1 cup papaya chunks
- 1 tablespoon freshly grated ginger
- 2 tablespoons fresh lime juice
- 1 tablespoon maple syrup
- 2 cups coconut water
- 2 cups plain soda water
- Ice cubes
- Pineapple wedges for garnish

Preparation:
1. In a blender, combine pineapple chunks, papaya chunks, grated ginger, lime juice, and maple syrup.

2. Blend until smooth.

3. Strain the tropical mixture to ensure a smooth liquid.

4. Fill serving glasses with ice cubes.

5. Pour the tropical blend equally into each glass.

6. Add coconut water and plain soda water, adjusting to your taste preference.

7. Stir gently to combine.

8. Garnish each glass with a pineapple wedge.

9. Serve immediately and enjoy the vibrant flavors of the Tropical Ginger Zinger!

Nutritional Information:

- Serving Size: 1 glass
- Calories: 70 kcal
- Total Fat: 0.2g
- Saturated Fat: 0g
- Cholesterol: 0mg
- Sodium: 30mg
- Total Carbohydrates: 17g
- Dietary Fiber: 1.5g
- Sugars: 13g
- Protein: 0.8g

Minty Citrus Splash

Ingredients:

- 1 cup fresh orange juice
- 1 cup fresh grapefruit juice
- 2 tablespoons fresh lemon juice

- 1 tablespoon maple syrup
- 1/4 cup fresh mint leaves
- 2 cups cold water
- 2 cups lemon-lime flavored sparkling water
- Ice cubes
- Citrus slices and mint sprigs for garnish

Preparation:

1. In a pitcher, combine orange juice, grapefruit juice, lemon juice, maple syrup, and fresh mint leaves.

2. Stir well to mix the flavors.

3. Fill serving glasses with ice cubes.

4. Pour the citrus-mint mixture equally into each glass.

5. Add cold water and lemon-lime flavored sparkling water, adjusting to your taste preference.

6. Stir gently to combine.

7. Garnish each glass with citrus slices and mint sprigs.

8. Serve immediately and revel in the Minty Citrus Splash!

Nutritional Information:

- Serving Size: 1 glass
- Calories: 60 kcal
- Total Fat: 0.2g
- Saturated Fat: 0g
- Cholesterol: 0mg
- Sodium: 18mg
- Total Carbohydrates: 15g
- Dietary Fiber: 1g
- Sugars: 11g

- Protein: 0.8g

Lavender Lemon Fizz

Ingredients:
- 1 tablespoon dried culinary lavender
- 1 cup hot water
- 2 tablespoons honey
- 1/4 cup fresh lemon juice
- 2 cups cold water
- 2 cups plain tonic water
- Ice cubes
- Lemon slices and lavender sprigs for garnish

Preparation:
1. Steep the dried culinary lavender in hot water for 10-15 minutes to create lavender tea. Strain and discard the lavender.
2. Allow the lavender tea to cool to room temperature.
3. In a pitcher, combine lavender tea, honey, fresh lemon juice, and cold water. Stir well.
4. Fill serving glasses with ice cubes.
5. Pour the lavender-lemon mixture equally into each glass.
6. Top each glass with plain tonic water and stir gently.
7. Garnish with lemon slices and lavender sprigs.
8. Serve immediately and relish the floral notes of the Lavender Lemon Fizz!

Nutritional Information:
- Serving Size: 1 glass
- Calories: 45 kcal
- Total Fat: 0g
- Saturated Fat: 0g
- Cholesterol: 0mg
- Sodium: 20mg
- Total Carbohydrates: 12g
- Dietary Fiber: 0.5g
- Sugars: 9g
- Protein: 0g

Ginger Mint Refresher

Ingredients:
- 2 tablespoons fresh ginger, grated
- 1/4 cup fresh mint leaves
- 2 tablespoons maple syrup
- 2 tablespoons fresh lime juice
- 2 cups cold water
- 2 cups ginger-flavored kombucha
- Ice cubes
- Lime wedges and mint sprigs for garnish

Preparation:
1. In a blender, combine grated ginger, mint leaves, maple syrup, and fresh lime juice.
2. Blend until smooth.

3. In a pitcher, mix the ginger-mint blend with cold water.

4. Fill serving glasses with ice cubes.

5. Pour the ginger-mint mixture equally into each glass.

6. Top each glass with ginger-flavored kombucha and stir gently.

7. Garnish with lime wedges and mint sprigs.

8. Serve immediately and enjoy the invigorating taste of the Ginger Mint Refresher!

Nutritional Information:

- Serving Size: 1 glass
- Calories: 35 kcal
- Total Fat: 0g
- Saturated Fat: 0g
- Cholesterol: 0mg
- Sodium: 8mg
- Total Carbohydrates: 9g
- Dietary Fiber: 0.5g
- Sugars: 7g
- Protein: 0g

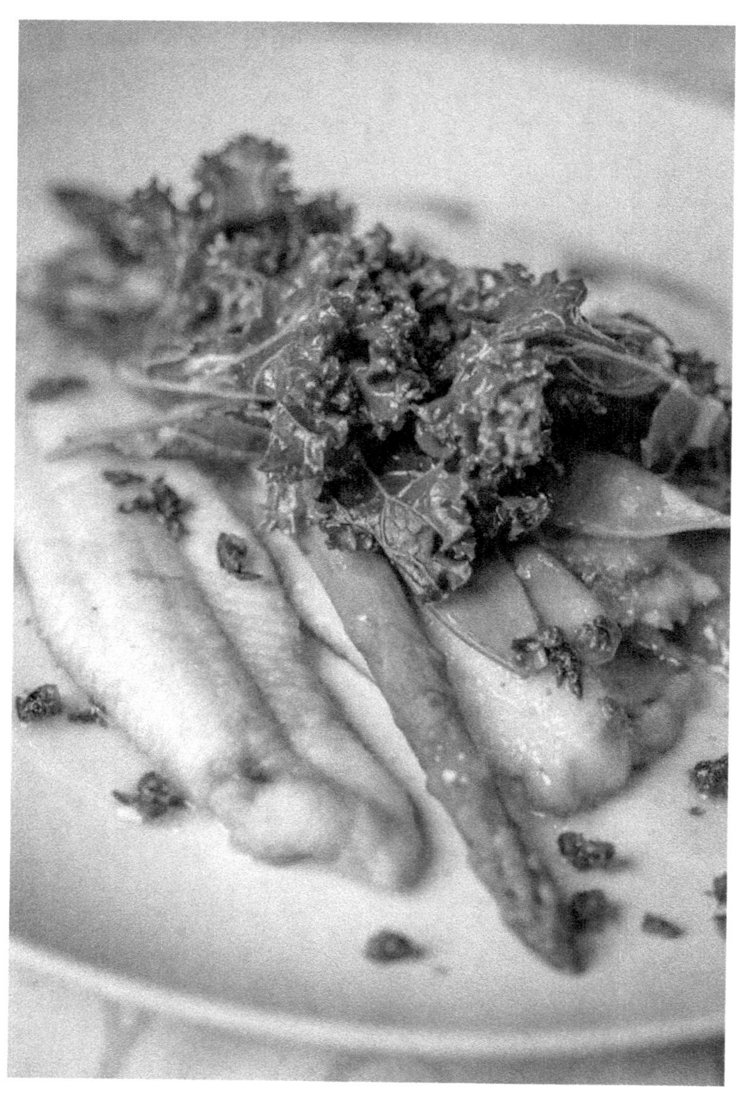

CONCLUSION

Embracing a Flavorful Low FODMAP Lifestyle

Welcome, everyone, to the journey of embracing a flavorful Low FODMAP lifestyle. Whether you're dealing with irritable bowel syndrome (IBS) or simply looking to improve your digestive health, adopting a Low FODMAP diet can be a game-changer. In this comprehensive guide, we'll explore what FODMAPs are, why a Low FODMAP lifestyle can be beneficial, and how to make the transition while still enjoying delicious and satisfying meals.

Understanding FODMAPs:

FODMAPs, which stands for Fermentable Oligosaccharides, Disaccharides, Monosaccharides, and Polyols, are short-chain carbohydrates that can ferment in the gut, leading to digestive discomfort for some individuals. High FODMAP foods include various fruits, vegetables, dairy products, grains, and sweeteners.

The Low FODMAP Approach:

The Low FODMAP diet involves reducing the intake of specific FODMAPs to alleviate digestive symptoms. This typically includes avoiding or limiting certain fruits, vegetables, dairy products, grains, and sweeteners during the initial phase. Finding trigger meals and progressively reintroducing them is the aim in order to ascertain each person's threshold for each food.

Building a Flavorful Low FODMAP Plate:

Contrary to popular belief, a Low FODMAP lifestyle doesn't mean sacrificing flavor. In fact, it's an opportunity to explore a wide range of delicious and nutritious foods. Here's how to build a flavorful Low FODMAP plate:

1. Protein:

  - Focus on lean meats, poultry, fish, and tofu.

  - Experiment with herbs, spices, and low FODMAP marinades for added flavor.

2. Vegetables:

  - Choose low FODMAP options such as spinach, zucchini, carrots, and bell peppers.

  - Use fresh herbs, garlic-infused oil, and ginger to enhance taste.

3. Fruits:

  - Opt for berries, kiwi, and citrus fruits in moderation.

  - Incorporate these fruits into snacks or desserts for a sweet touch.

4. Grains:

  - Select gluten-free grains like rice, quinoa, and oats.

  - Explore alternative flours like rice flour or almond flour for baking.

5. Dairy:

- Choose lactose-free or lactose-reduced dairy products.

- Experiment with non-dairy alternatives like almond or coconut milk.

6. Sweeteners:

- Use small amounts of maple syrup or stevia instead of high FODMAP sweeteners.

- Explore the world of natural sweeteners like cinnamon and vanilla.

Navigating Social Situations:

Adopting a Low FODMAP lifestyle doesn't mean missing out on social gatherings or dining out.The following advice can help you handle these circumstances:

1. Communication:

- Communicate your dietary needs to friends, family, and restaurants in advance.

2. Menu Exploration:

- Choose dishes that are likely to be Low FODMAP or ask for modifications.

3. BYO (Bring Your Own):

- Consider bringing your own Low FODMAP dish to ensure a safe and satisfying meal.

Embracing a flavorful Low FODMAP lifestyle is not only manageable but also rewarding. By understanding FODMAPs, making informed food choices, and experimenting with flavors, you can create a diverse and delicious menu that supports your digestive health. Remember, it's a journey of self-discovery, and finding the right balance for your body is key. Here's to a flavorful and fulfilling Low FODMAP experience!

Exploring Further Low FODMAP Culinary Adventures

Welcome, adventurous cooks, to the world of Low FODMAP culinary exploration! If you've been navigating the intricate landscape of FODMAPs (Fermentable Oligosaccharides, Disaccharides, Monosaccharides, and Polyols) and have successfully embarked on your Low FODMAP journey, it's time to take your culinary adventures to the next level.

In this culinary expedition, we'll delve deeper into the realm of Low FODMAP ingredients, discovering new flavors, textures, and innovative combinations that will elevate your dishes to extraordinary heights. So, fasten your aprons, sharpen your knives, and let's dive into the world of delectable Low FODMAP creations!

Exploring the Low FODMAP Pantry:

1. Grains and Alternatives:
   - Beyond rice and quinoa, experiment with lesser-known grains like millet, sorghum, and buckwheat. These grains add unique textures and flavors to your meals while staying within the Low FODMAP guidelines.

2. Herbs and Spices:
   - Elevate your dishes with an array of fresh herbs such as chives, basil, and cilantro. Experiment with infused oils or make your own herb blends to add a burst of flavor without triggering FODMAPs.

3. Proteins:
   - Venture beyond the usual chicken and beef. Try incorporating seafood like shrimp, salmon, or even calamari for a delightful change. Tofu and tempeh can also be excellent plant-based protein options.

4. Vegetables:
   - While certain vegetables are off-limits, there are plenty of exciting options to explore. Roasted bell peppers, zucchini noodles, and grilled eggplant can bring variety and color to your dishes.

5. Dairy Alternatives:
   - Experiment with lactose-free or Low FODMAP alternatives like almond milk, lactose-free yogurt, and aged cheeses. These substitutes maintain the creaminess and richness in your recipes.

Cooking Techniques and Innovations:

1. Infused Oils and Vinegars:
   - Create your own infused oils with garlic-infused oil or rosemary-infused olive oil for added depth of flavor. Balsamic and rice vinegar can also be used to enhance dishes without introducing FODMAPs.

2. Grilling and Roasting:
   - Explore the bold flavors achieved through grilling and roasting. Char-grilled meats, vegetables, and even fruits can add a delightful smokiness to your Low FODMAP creations.

3. Homemade Sauces and Condiments:
   - Craft your own Low FODMAP sauces and condiments using safe ingredients. From a zesty tomato-free marinara to a tangy BBQ sauce, the possibilities are endless.

4. Fresh and Fermented:
   - Incorporate the freshness of citrus fruits and the tang of pickled vegetables to lift the flavors in your dishes. Experiment with lacto-fermented foods like sauerkraut and kimchi for a probiotic boost.

Congratulations, culinary explorers! By expanding your Low FODMAP horizons, you've unlocked a world of delicious possibilities. Remember, creativity is your greatest ally in the kitchen. So, continue to experiment, adapt, and savor the joys of crafting flavorful, Low

FODMAP masterpieces that delight your taste buds and nourish your well-being. Happy cooking!

Acknowledgments and Resources

I would like to express my gratitude to the individuals and organizations that have contributed to the development of resources related to the Low FODMAP diet. Their dedication to providing accurate and helpful information has been invaluable in supporting individuals managing gastrointestinal conditions. We acknowledge their efforts in raising awareness and improving the quality of life for those following a Low FODMAP lifestyle.

Resources for Low FODMAP Information:
1. Monash University FODMAP App:
   - Monash University is a pioneer in FODMAP research, and their app provides comprehensive information on foods that are low or high in FODMAPs. It includes a searchable database and helpful tools for individuals following a Low FODMAP diet.
   - Website: [Monash University FODMAP App](https://www.monashfodmap.com/)
2. The FODMAP Friendly Program:
   - The FODMAP Friendly Program certifies food products that meet their low FODMAP standards. Their

certification helps individuals easily identify suitable products when grocery shopping.

- Website: [FODMAP Friendly](https://fodmapfriendly.com/)

3. International Foundation for Gastrointestinal Disorders (IFFGD):

- IFFGD provides educational resources on various gastrointestinal disorders, including information on the Low FODMAP diet. Their website offers articles, webinars, and support for individuals managing digestive health.

- Website: [IFFGD](https://aboutgimotility.org/)

4. Beyond FODMAPs:

- Beyond FODMAPs is a platform that offers recipes, meal plans, and lifestyle tips for those following a Low FODMAP diet. It aims to make the journey more enjoyable and diverse for individuals with dietary restrictions.

- Website: [Beyond FODMAPs](https://www.beyondfodmaps.com/)

5. The Monash University Low FODMAP Dietitian Directory:

- For personalized guidance, the Monash University Low FODMAP Dietitian Directory helps individuals find registered dietitians experienced in the Low FODMAP diet. Consulting a dietitian can enhance the effectiveness of the dietary approach.

- Website: [Monash FODMAP Dietitian Directory](https://www.monashfodmap.com/blog/find-a-dietitian/)

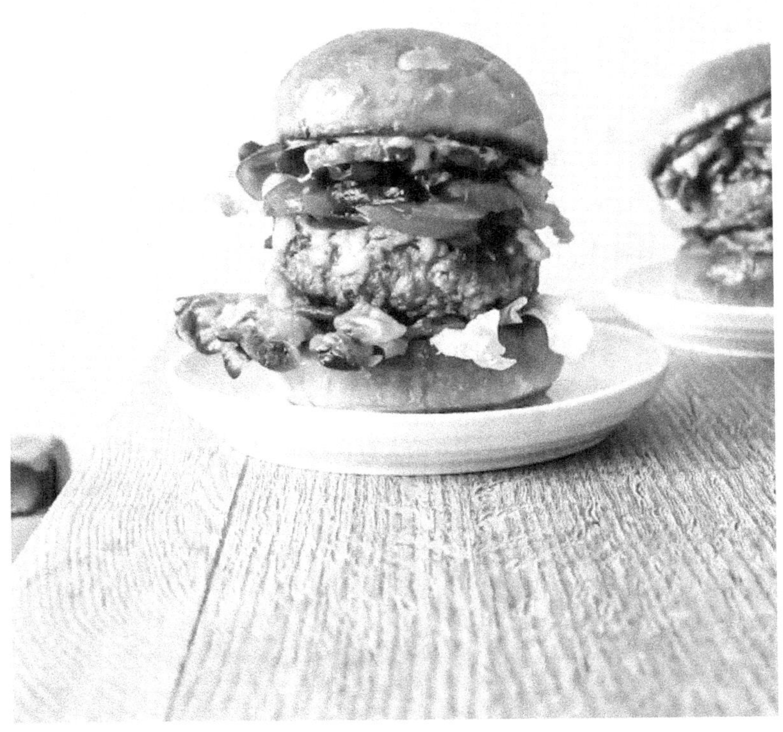

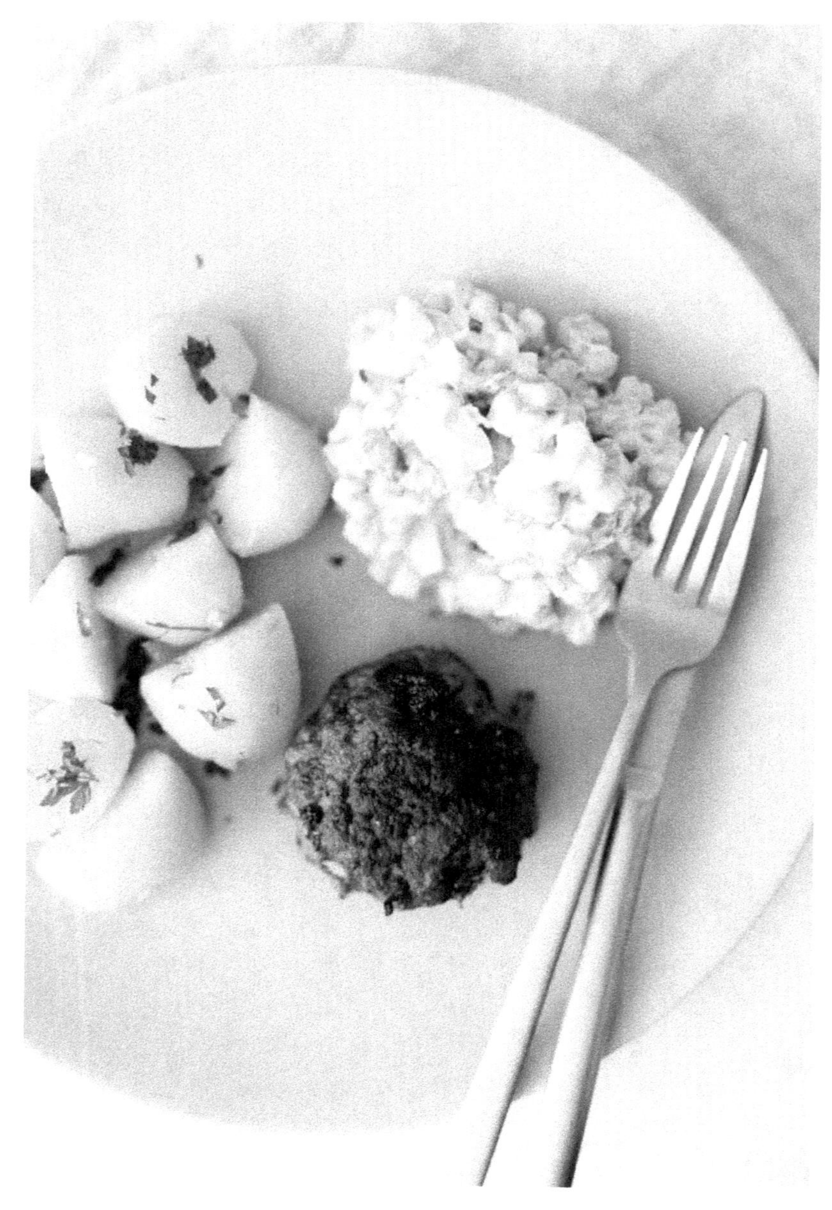